FUND-RAISING
for Animal Care Organizations

Edited by Julie Miller Dowling

Made possible through a generous grant
from the Munder Family Foundation

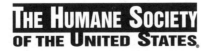

HUMANE SOCIETY
U N I V E R S I T Y

Julie Miller Dowling is a former editor of
Animal Sheltering magazine and a consultant
for The Humane Society of the United States.
She is the author of the forthcoming manual
How to Form a Humane Organization.

First edition
ISBN 0-9748400-2-5
Library of Congress Cataloging-in Publication Data

Fund-Raising for Animal Care Organizations / edited by Julie Miller Dowling.
      p. cm. – (Shelter management series)
   "The Humane Society of the United States."
   "Made possible through a generous grant from the Munder Family Foundation."
   Includes bibliographical references.
   ISBN 0-9748400-2-5
   1. Animal welfare–United States–Societies, etc.–Finance. 2. Fund raising–United States.
   I. Miller Dowling, Julie. II. Humane Society of the United States. III. Series.
   HV4763.F85 2005
   636.08'32'0681–dc22

                          2005002811

Printed in the United States of America

Humane Society Press
An affiliate of The Humane Society of the United States
2100 L Street, NW
Washington, D.C. 20037
humanesocietypress.org

Permissions

Table 3.3, Table 3.4, the Code of Ethical Principles and Standards (chapter 4), the Donor Bill of Rights (chapter 4), and Principles of the E-Donor Bill of Rights (chapter 12): Copyright 2004, *Advancing Philanthropy*, Association of Fundraising Professionals (AFP), formerly NSFRE, all rights reserved. Reprinted with permission.

Table 5.1, Conflict of Interest (chapter 4), Ten Basic Responsibilities of Nonprofit Boards, Individual Board Member Responsibilities, and Personal Characteristics to Consider (all chapter 5), Getting Everyone to Get Along (appendix C) reprinted with permission from *www.boardsource.org*. For more information about BoardSource, formerly the National Center for Nonprofit Boards, visit *www.boardsource.org* or call 800-883-6262. BoardSource © 2005. Text may not be reproduced without written permission from BoardSource.

Table 3.2: Center on Philanthropy at Indiana University, 2004. Reprinted with permission.

The Ten Rules of e-Philanthropy that Every Nonprofit Must Know (chapter 12): reprinted with permission from the ePhilanthropyFoundation.Org © 2001, 2002.

Figure 8.1 reprinted with permission from The Foundation Center, *Foundation Giving Trends*, 2004. Based on sample of 1,005 larger U.S. foundations.

Figure 1.1 and Table 9.1 reprinted with permission from Giving USA 2004, Giving USA Foundation™, AAFRC Trust for Philanthropy.

Table 6.1 reprinted with special permission of Independent Sector. *www.IndependentSector.org*.

Table 2.1 reprinted with permission from Society of Animal Welfare Administrators, 2003 Survey.

Table 7.1 and Table 7.2 reprinted with permission from Vertis Customer Focus.

Other Books in the Humane Society Press Shelter Management Series

Volunteer Management for Animal Care Organizations
by Betsy McFarland

Editor's Note

This project was made possible through a generous grant from the Munder Family Foundation. *Fund-Raising for Animal Care Organizations* is the second book in the Humane Society Press Shelter Management Series funded by Lee Munder, who has recognized the need for hands-on books tailored to the animal care community, on fund-raising in particular. The Humane Society of the United States (HSUS) and I thank him for his generous support and thoughtful leadership throughout this project.

Many animal care experts lent their time and talents to this project. Special thanks go to my coauthors, who contributed their broad knowledge and experience in fund-raising for animal causes:

Judith A. Calhoun (chapters 9 and 10)
Vice President of Development/Community Relations
Dumb Friends League
Denver, Colorado

Vincent F. Connelly (chapter 7)
President, Connelly and Associates Fund-raising LLC
Baltimore, Maryland

Caryn Ginsberg (chapter 2)
Co-founder, Priority Ventures Group
Arlington, Virginia

Karen Medicus (chapters 1, 3, 5, 6, and 11)
Director, Imagine Humane
(A project of ASPCA and PETsMART Charities)
Austin, Texas

M. Christie Smith (chapter 4)
Executive Director, Potter League for Animals
Newport, Rhode Island

Alice Tracy, Ph.D. (chapter 8)
Director, Foundation Relations
The Humane Society of the United States
Washington, D.C.

I wrote chapter 12.

The HSUS, my coauthors, and I are grateful to the following reviewers: Diane Allevato (executive director, Marin Humane Society, Novato, California), Jennifer Bahlmann (board president, West Suburban Humane Society, Chicago, Illinois), David Gies (executive director of Animal Assistance Foundation, Denver, Colorado), Gordon Kromberg (board member, Animal Welfare League of Alexandria, Virginia), Laura Maloney (executive director, Louisiana SPCA, New Orleans, Louisiana), Bill Sturtevant (vice president for Principal Gifts, University of Illinois Foundation, Champaign, Illinois), and Jim Tedford (account director, Grizzard Communications, Knoxville, Tennessee).

Thanks go, too, to the organizations that provided samples from their own fund-raising programs: Maryland SPCA (Baltimore, Maryland), Los Angeles County Animal Care Foundation (Los Angeles, California), Dumb Friends League (Denver, Colorado), and Animal Welfare League of Alexandria.

This manual would not have been possible without the contributions of staff at The HSUS. Traci Bryant, Betsy McFarland, and Kate Pullen served as project managers. Carol Baker, Tom Knox, Beth McNulty, Paula Jaworski, Robert Roop, Ph.D., Andrew Rowan, Ph.D., and Deborah Salem were also most helpful.

—Julie Miller Dowling

Contents

Figures

Tables

Chapter 1

Getting Started: How to Set Yourself Up for Fund-Raising Success

A for-profit's mission is to create as much value for its stockholders as possible, within the constraints of society. The nonprofit's mission is to create as much value for society as possible, within the constraints of its money.

—Peter W. Likins, president, University of Arizona (Jensen 1999, 2).

Your organization works hard every day to improve the lives of animals and people in your community. The public should appreciate that and place bags of money at your door to help your cause. And the public should do it happily, without any prompting on your part. After all, you are busy enough with spay/neuter campaigns, adoptions, humane education, public outreach, pet-behavior counseling, animal rescues, and lobbying. Certainly, you cannot be expected to actively raise funds, too!

Alas, as you no doubt have discovered, the world does not work as it should. People do not part with their money readily; they need to be enticed to open their wallets for a cause—no matter how worthy. So you and your peers in the animal care community face a catch-22: you need money to carry out the (literally) life-saving work you do, but you cannot seem to find time to plan anything beyond the occasional dog walk and hastily produced "how to donate" link on your web site. Fund-raising is a back-burner project that never makes it to the front burner.

The result? Your organization's programs never sizzle. Your animal care organization is so busy putting out small fires, the result of inadequate planning and funding, that it simply can't fulfill its principal goals or even its mission. If this statement makes you shift uncomfortably in your seat, then *Fund-Raising for Animal Care Organizations* is for you. In it you will discover how successfully planned fund-raising has helped hundreds of animal care organizations raise thousands of dollars for basic necessities and ambitious, innovative programs, and you will learn about the many types of fund-raising that can be channeled to meet the diverse needs of your organization.

But first you will need to take the first step—have an attitude adjustment. You need to view fund-raising not as a sideline project that you get to when you find time but as the center-stage program that fuels your organization. Do not be hesitant or shy about asking for money—you are a charity case! Remember the fund-raising mantra: "The key to giving is asking." To succeed, you simply cannot separate raising funds from operating an animal care organization. The success of the second depends on the success of the first.

Loose Change Is Not Enough

Not all fund-raising methods are equal. Setting up "please help" coin canisters inside a few local shops and sitting with a donation jar in front of a supermarket do not demand much planning or people power. But if you have tried raising money for your animal care organization this way, you likely have discovered that the pocket change of passersby cannot pay for operational expenses or innovative new projects.

What can pay for these essentials is a combination of the more sophisticated fund-raising methods, such as annual giving, major gifts, direct mail, grants, planned giving, special events, and capital campaigns. While these certainly demand more planning, people, resources, and follow-through, well-executed fund-raisers can bring in the larger and more consistent donations that allow your organization to stop treading water and instead serve as an effective lifeguard for animals in your community.

It Is Worth the Effort

By prioritizing fund-raising, busy organizations have found the time to develop a strategic development plan and raise enough resources to expand beyond basic programs. Here are just a few examples of the fund-raising successes realized by local animal care organizations.

- Careful planning and creative thinking earned the Fox Valley Humane Society $25,000 at its innovative "special event" held a few years ago. Guests at the "Mystery Made to Order" event were encouraged to help solve the "kidnapping" of an opera-singing golden retriever named Basso Profundo Pooch while enjoying an elegant dinner. Not only did the event bring in substantial funds, it also gleaned a priceless contact. One of the attendees, who happened to be the executive director of the Wisconsin Committee to Prevent Child Abuse, was so impressed with the event that she agreed to combine efforts for the following year's fund-raiser and launch a joint educational campaign focusing on the link between animal abuse and child abuse.

- Through dedicated and skilled volunteer support, the Anne Arundel County (Maryland) SPCA raised $40,000 via its used-vehicle donation program. The program was run by one dedicated volunteer, who picked up vehicles from donors' residences, cleaned and repaired the cars, placed "for sale" ads, and negotiated the final sale.

- Developing relationships with corporate contributors brought the Atlanta Humane Society (AHS) big bucks. It teamed up with the Atlanta Braves to produce a calendar featuring burly ball players and cuddly animal centerfolds. Sales of the popular calendar generated $53,000 and plenty of visibility for AHS, and the Braves management considered the cooperative effort a great way to promote the team's philanthropic efforts.

- Taking the time to create and manage an appealing, user-friendly web site generated thousands of dollars for the Humane Society of Rochester and Monroe County (New York). Site visitors see instantly how to donate or become a member online. The site also links to the shelter's online gift shop, where people can make donations or purchase shelter T-shirts, dining discount coupon booklets, and memorial bricks for the shelter's entrance walkway.

Wait—Not So Fast

Hungry for money to fuel their programs, many organizations attempt to replicate these kinds of fund-raising success stories before developing the foundation necessary for success. Why is it so critical that you devote scarce time and resources to plan and run your fund-raisers? According to The Center on Philanthropy at Indiana University (2004b), charitable organizations in the United States receive more than $240 billion in contributions annually. The environment/animal sub-sector receives 2.9 percent or $6.95 billion of that $240 billion (Figure 1.1). The percentage received by animal care organizations could grow over time if they were to professionalize their programs and outreach.

Figure 1.1

2003 Contributions by Source (in billions)

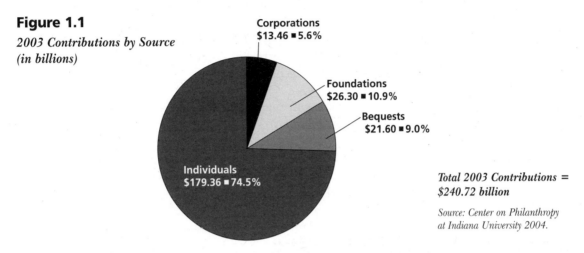

Corporations
$13.46 ■ 5.6%

Foundations
$26.30 ■ 10.9%

Bequests
$21.60 ■ 9.0%

Individuals
$179.36 ■ 74.5%

Total 2003 Contributions = $240.72 billion

Source: Center on Philanthropy at Indiana University 2004.

So why not just rush out and grab your rightful share? In reality, poorly run fund-raising programs can end up costing you more than you bring in. Need more convincing? Take a look at these real-world fund-raising disasters:

■ One local animal care organization was left in disarray when the disgruntled employee who controlled the organization's web site quit, taking the web site and all fund-raising records with her. She then started another organization in the same area. Had the original organization invested in creating a dependable fund-raising tracking system accessible and managed by more than one individual, it could have avoided this costly catastrophe.

■ Eager for "easy" money, an animal care organization accepted a socialite's proposal to chair a gala event to benefit the organization. The organization had an unwilling board, a poor committee structure, and no money to pay for the event. Its leadership just assumed that the socialite would cover the up-front costs necessary to create the event; she was given the reins to steer the project but no policies or process to follow. Later, the organization's director was shocked to discover that the socialite had signed contracts—in the name of the organization—for a band, the most exclusive hotel in town, champagne, and a sit-down dinner. She even asked to set up a bank account in her name to receive all the donations. By jumping at the chance for "free" money, the organization learned too late how dangerous it is to rely on offers that sound too good to be true.

■ An animal care organization received a large gift from an individual to build a spay/neuter clinic that bore her name. Because donor records were maintained poorly, information about that "major-gift" project was eventually lost and forgotten. The new management, which had no details about the gift or the donor, decided to take the name off the building. The donor was still living in the area and was planning to leave half of her substantial estate to the organization. Luckily, the new management discovered its error before the donor found out about its plan. Strong, long-term donor relations depend on strong, long-term donor record systems.

A less dramatic but possibly bigger mistake many organizations make is to go after money for special projects without first ensuring their long-term sustainability. Committing revenues from supporters to underwrite a new project or enhanced service may simply result in robbing Peter (kennel-cleaning staff) to pay Paul (innovative spay/neuter mobile clinic). Make sure that you can guarantee general operation funds to protect basic existing services before soliciting donations earmarked for popular but optional new projects.

Starting on the Right Footing

The key to increasing donations, fulfilling goals, and avoiding calamities is to launch your fund-raising program from a firm, reliable base. Your organization must first possess or create the solid policies, people, programs, and plans needed for successful fund-raising. Take a look at this checklist to make sure your organization has what it takes.

☐ Our organization has and actively uses a current, detailed, customized, workable strategic plan on which to base our development (fund-raising) plan.

☐ Our organization has a reliable, integrated, comprehensive record-keeping system to manage our programs.

☐ Our organization produces detailed, accurate financial records that enable our leaders to monitor and understand our organization's current and future financial needs.

☐ Our organization's staff, volunteers, and leadership have a clear sense of our organization's mission, vision, and constituency (supporters and service users).

☐ Our organization's board of directors understands and is committed to its roles and responsibilities, including fund-raising.

☐ Our organization's staff, volunteers, and board cooperate and communicate effectively to advance the mission of our organization.

☐ Our organization understands the needs and expectations of our community and customizes programs and projects to meet those needs.

☐ Our organization is aware of the other local animal-related organizations and strives to cooperate with them without duplicating services.

If you were able to check all these boxes, you are well on your way to creating a top-notch fund-raising program. If you have left a few boxes unchecked, this manual can help you bridge those gaps.

Different fund-raising methods can help your animal care organization bring in needed income. Each method produces different amounts of money at different rates. Some fund-raising initiatives take months or years to develop, while others can be completed in a few weeks. Each technique has its pros and cons: grant money, for example, can be a terrific boost to a new program, but it is no substitute for the small, steady trickle of monthly donations that your organization can use as unrestricted operational money.

To develop the best way to approach these fund-raising methods, it may help to play a game of darts at your local watering hole. Visualizing a dartboard can help you understand how the best fund-raising strategies unfold. "At the center is your board of directors," explains Robert DeMartinis, a fund-raising consultant and guide to *About.com*'s Nonprofit Charitable Organizations. "In separate concentric circles moving away from the center are staff and volunteers, vendors, community businesses and individuals, and finally foundations" (DeMartinis, n.d., 1). As you expand your fund-raising programs and incorporate new methods, make sure you tap the talents and wallets of those closest to your organization. Remember, too, that big givers come from your pool of small givers.

Why Do Donors Give?

Donors give for many reasons: their interests match your organization's mission; they want to be seen as leaders in the community; they see your organization as financially sound and reputable; they want to make a difference in the world; they feel a sense of gratitude to your organization; or they have a strong relationship with someone in your organization.

Why People Give

- People give to people.
- People give money because they want to.
- People don't give unless or until they are asked.
- People don't give large donations unless they are asked for large donations.
- People give to opportunities, not to needs.
- People give to success, not to distress.
- People give to causes that improve their "quality of life."
- People give because they want to "make a difference."
- People give because they want to be involved in something bigger than themselves.
- People give because of an "attitude of gratitude."

Types of Giving

Annual Giving
Acquiring new donors (such as those who use agency services) can help your organization broaden its base. Typical activities to generate first-time annual giving—also known in the industry as "acquisition"—include direct mail, telethons, donor clubs, telephone gifts, special events, and media. This is the primary fund-raising method used to broaden support, upgrade giving levels, and provide operating support for ongoing programs.

"Repeat annual giving" is what provides financial stability. As donor commitment grows, you build a strong donor base and begin to encourage donors to consider larger gifts and deeper involvement in your organization. Typical activities to generate this type of giving include personal contact, letters, and phone calls. Fund-raising is friend-raising, and this is where you begin to expand your circle of friends. Workplace giving campaigns can facilitate recurrent giving as well through payroll deductions and direct contribution via United Way, Combined Federal Campaign, or similar campaigns for state employees.

Direct mail, another form of annual giving, is covered in chapter 7.

Major Giving
The process of obtaining larger gifts focuses more on relationships than it does on money. To develop major gifts, the organization must match donors' interests with the organization's needs. Typical activities to generate this type of giving include personal contact, letters, and phone calls. Individuals, corporations, and foundations are involved in fund-raising at this level (see chapter 6).

Capital Giving
This is an intensive, organized fund-raising effort to secure donations for specific capital needs or projects. A capital campaign typically is executed within a specific time frame, usually more than one year. These large gifts can be considered "stretch gifts" for donors, so these donors are solicited only once (see chapter 11).

Planned Giving
As people age and retire, their capacity for making lifetime gifts grows. Donations through bequests, gifts of life insurance, and other types of life income and deferred gifts increase with asset accumulation. Typical vehicles for this type of giving may include wills, bequests, estate planning, insurance policies, and gift annuities (see chapter 9).

Table 1.1
Diversity of Income Sources for Animal Care Organizations

Shelter	1	2	3	4	5	6	7
Events	$63,000	$12,000	$20,000	$195,000	$20,000	$10,000	$25,000
Publications	$4,000						
Tag Sale	$4,000						
Donations		$70,000	$245,000	$140,000	$500,000	$150,000	$200,000
Canister Program		$1,000					
Bequests		$11,000	$20,000				
Interest/Dividends		$40,000	$1,000	$2,000	$10,000	$15,000	$4,000
Trusts/Foundations		$62,000					
Grants						$250,000	
Municipal Contract		$75,000					$140,000
Merchandise		$41,000	$60,000				
Catalogue Sales					$12,000		
Adoption Fees		$125,000		$15,000			$175,000
Service Fees			$50,000			$15,000	$12,000
Direct Mail	$18,000			$30,000			
Member Fees				$5,000	$10,000	$45,000	
Total	$89,000	$437,000	$396,000	$387,000	$552,000	$485,000	$556,000

Source: Data compiled from various animal shelter annual reports.

This list does not include all categories of giving. For example, other sources for funding can include income from rentals, sales/service (i.e., veterinary care and grooming), investment/endowment, and municipal contracts. Table 1.1, which provides an example of animal care organizations' diversity of income sources, shows that significant funds are available to such organizations. When creating a development plan, explore all possibilities and never close doors to any opportunity for increasing your financial growth and, ultimately, your program growth.

A successful fund development program integrates the types of giving to support the funding needs of your organization over the course of its lifetime. The appropriate mix of all of these types will depend on your organization's need for operating income, capital improvement, physical plant, income, and funds for special programs. Most organizations begin with annual giving programs to build their organizational friendships and develop a strong donor base to build depth. As you develop your fund-raising campaign, diversify the types of giving you seek and avoid focusing on one method over another. Even if you are not yet prepared to launch a major-gifts or capital campaign program, be sure to include the concept in your planning for long-term sustainability of your organization's funding needs.

Despite the billions donated to charities, fund-raising today remains a challenge for nonprofits that must compete for donor dollars in uncertain times. Although this manual cannot cover everything you need to know about fund-raising, it can give you the jump start you need to customize a development plan that works for your animal care organization, in your town, for your animals. If you need more information, see Resources for improving and expanding your fund-raising knowledge and programs.

Chapter 2

Finding Your Identity: How to Show Them What You've Got

Your friend in Sweet Town asks you to invest in her bakery. How do you decide whether to put your money into this venture? Of course, you want to find out whether you are likely to get a good return on your investment. Do you just assume that the bakery draws lots of customers and enjoys little competition, or do you expect your friend to provide facts and figures that prove her business is worthy of your investment? To ensure that your hard-earned money will not support a half-baked scheme, you need answers to these questions:

- What is the makeup of the population?
- What is the demand for bakery products?
- How has the bakery been doing to date? What are its strengths and weaknesses?
- What is special about this bakery compared to others in the community?
- How does the bakery create a unique impression to attract business?
- Does the facility itself appear clean and inviting to entice visitors?

It may be true that your friend bakes the best cakes in town, but if she has not done her homework to support her business, both of you will likely be disappointed in the results.

Showing Them What You've Got

Potential donors will ask similar questions of your animal care organization. Donors do not expect to gain financially from their contributions to your nonprofit cause, but they do expect a return on their investment. Foundations and donors want to make sure that their dollars will produce the most benefit possible for animals and the community. Corporate sponsors expect to generate a positive image and new business through their support of your cause.

If a donor dangled a $1,000 check in front of you and said, "I'd like to donate to a worthy animal-protection organization, but I need to make sure this money goes to the right one," how would you respond? Could you tell the donor exactly what sets your organization apart from other nonprofits and animal-related businesses? Could you explain how your services meet specific needs of the community? Could you demonstrate your organization's viability and the success of its programs? Successful fund-raising depends on your organization's responses to these kinds of queries.

To make sure your organization's marketing is up to today's fund-raising challenges, take a fresh look inside and out. Examine your community demographics and demands and find out what your target constituencies think about your organization. Evaluate your organization to make sure it is doing all it can to meet local needs and determine what makes it exceptional. Use this information to develop a niche and a positioning statement that shows donors what makes your organization special and worthy of their investment. (If you need help assessing your community and evaluating your organization, see appendix A.)

Defining your Niche

According to the Alliance for Nonprofit Management (n.d., n.p.), a professional association devoted to improving the management and governance capacity of nonprofits, the

> [I]ncreasing demand for a smaller pool of resources requires today's nonprofits to rethink how they do business, to compete where appropriate, to avoid duplicating existing comparable services, and to increase collaboration where possible.

Your animal care organization cannot stand back in the shadows if it wants to help animals, garner public backing, and earn financial support. Your community will not help you if it doesn't know you are there and cannot understand what sets you apart from other animal-related organizations. Even if your organization is the only animal-protection agency in town, you still compete with other nonprofit organizations, pet stores, veterinarians, and breed placement groups, among others, for attention and dollars. Nationally, you are up against similar organizations seeking funding from foundations and donors. Table 2.1 breaks down total development revenues for animal shelters by fund-raising type. It shows that special events generally bring in about the same amount of money, regardless of the organization's size, while direct mail, annual gifts, and other types of fund-raising in which you ask for a specific gift generally bring in more money as the organization grows.

Table 2.1

Total Development Revenues for Animal Shelters, by Fund-Raising Type

	Less than $1 million	$1–$2.9 million	$3–$4.9 million	$5 million or more	All Organizations
Direct Mail	$73,000	$117,000	$454,000	$3,236,000	$620,000
Annual Gifts	$106,000	$180,000	$750,000	$1,180,000	$398,000
Special Events	$129,000	$388,000	$288,000	$482,000	$287,000
Other (memorials, foundations, etc.)	$88,000	$250,000	$697,000	$1,347,000	$436,000

Source: Society of Animal Welfare Administrators 2003.

Your organization needs to identify what makes it special and show this to the public and funders. Can you spot your organization's niche? Review these examples to see if your organization can claim any of the following:

- "We provide the best information on helping people and animals enjoy living together in homes and throughout the community."

- "We offer subsidized spay/neuter and veterinary services to low-income individuals to reduce the number of sick, unwanted animals and to promote responsible pet care."

- "We deliver outstanding client service and quality care that attracts people to the shelter, motivates them to return, prompts them to tell others, and encourages them to donate."

It is not always easy to boil down your organization's many programs and projects into a concise phrase that outsiders can digest. If you are having trouble identifying your niche or selecting one to establish, try a mix of these methods:

■ Use your mission and vision statements to guide you, but do not let them limit your creativity in defining a role where you can truly serve your community and flourish financially.

■ Review or determine your community's most pressing needs. Can your organization address these? If not, what changes can it make to tackle these challenges?

■ Participate with your community's local support resources—such as your local or state association for nonprofit organizations—that provide management support to nonprofit organizations.

■ Compare your animal care organization objectively and constructively to other local organizations helping animals. Do you serve certain populations, offer unique programs, or have special strengths that would help you differentiate your organization from them?

■ Investigate how animal care organizations around the country are succeeding. Can you find examples in *Animal Sheltering* magazine (*www.AnimalSheltering.org*), at conferences, or through networking that identify new approaches you can focus on?

■ Use research and focus groups to learn what your community, clients, and current donors think. What distinct role do they believe you play or could play in the community? How would they react to options you may be considering? (Market research companies have been generous and supportive in sponsoring focus groups in many communities. For more information on market research companies, focus groups, and polling, see appendix A.)

If you are having difficulty honing in on potential areas of distinction, analyze each of your programs individually. The MacMillan Matrix, developed by Ian MacMillan of the Wharton School of Business, can help you assess whether your programs fit your organization. This "strategy grid" (at *www.allianceonline.org*) helps nonprofits address these important questions:

■ Are we the best organization to provide this service?

■ Is competition good for our clients?

■ Are we spreading ourselves too thin, without the capacity to sustain ourselves?

■ Should we work cooperatively with another organization to provide services?

For more about the MacMillan Matrix, see Resources.

Staking Out Your Position Statement

After you have defined your niche, you are ready to communicate your distinctiveness to the public through a "positioning statement" that:

- captures the main view you want your constituents to hold about your organization

- summarizes the ideal reputation that you would like for your shelter

- motivates your audience to take action and become involved

- delivers a memorable, succinct, distinct, and focused message

To craft your positioning statement, look at the niche you have defined. How will it benefit your community? How will people feel about that benefit? Think about what you would want one community member to say to another about your organization. You won't necessarily use the statement word-for-word in your communications, but it should reflect how you would like to be portrayed. For example:

- "Anytown Shelter is the source in our community for the advice and assistance I trust to handle important decisions on living with animals."

- "The ABC Spay/Neuter Group reduces suffering by helping people in need access affordable veterinary services for their animals to prevent disease, birth of unwanted animals, and relinquishment."

- "*Www.xyzhumanesociety.org* is a one-stop resource I can count on to find answers to questions regarding pets and wildlife in my county."

Consider developing a positioning statement for different stakeholders or programs. Just be sure that each customized statement reflects the general reputation and mission of your organization.

Here is an example of a positioning statement for an animal care organization's capital campaign: "A state-of-the-art animal shelter with progressive programs will improve lives by raising the bar for animal care in our shelter and in our community." Note how this statement not only includes the benefit of the new facility but also reinforces the image of the shelter as the leader in defining and delivering quality animal care in the community.

Your positioning statement is not a catchy slogan or slick ad, so don't worry about writing perfect text. Instead, think of your positioning statement as the anchor for all your other communications. All slogans, taglines, messages, and imagery should be developed or refined to reflect and strengthen the positioning.

For example, if you are trying to present a serious, professional image, avoid cute cartoon images that detract from your ultimate goal. Review all in-shelter signs, mail, web sites, brochures, ads, newsletters, and other forms of communication to ensure that you are consistently reinforcing the positioning verbally and visually.

Your organization will use this position statement along with your mission statement and other internal documents to develop its "case statement." This statement bundles together in one attractive, neat document all that is important for potential donors to know about your organization: its mission, history, goals, objectives, plans, programs, budget, leadership, and staff. You will use information from your case statement in virtually all of your publications and fund-raising appeals, from newsletters to grant proposals (for more on what goes into a case statement, see chapter 11).

When you have positioned your organization successfully, people understand and recognize what you are and what you do in the community. Assuming the position statement and case statement accurately reflect your organization, donations are more likely to come your way.

Putting on Your Best Face

Mr. Rich Moola loves animals and has some money to give. He first visits the Sorry State Humane Society's sheltering facility, which greets him with unpleasant smells, loud barking, a dripping ceiling, and an invisible staff. He picks up the organization's few tattered outreach and solicitation materials, noticing that they were printed on cheap paper using an old typewriter (which isn't equipped with "spell-check").

Mr. Moola crosses the bridge into the next town, where smiling volunteers welcome him to the Happy Times SPCA's clean, bright facility. He picks up colorful, reader-friendly education materials that he recalls seeing at a variety of public venues. Before leaving, he makes a mental note to ask his wife about adopting the adorable, purring tabby he visited in the shelter's "get acquainted" room.

Now Mr. Moola has a decision to make: which organization should get his money? At first glance the first organization appears more deserving because its situation is so dire and its needs are so great. But Mr. Moola is a savvy donor who wants to make sure the money he gives is used appropriately. He feels bad for Sorry State Humane Society, but he's not sure the faltering organization will even be around in the coming years. He's also concerned about the way the organization is managed—if it can't manage to have someone greet a visitor, and it can't manage to spell words correctly, then how can it manage to spend his money wisely?

Happy Times SPCA, on the other hand, obviously benefits from generous supporters. But Mr. Moola is drawn to the organization's success—successful spay/neuter program, successful volunteer support, successful adoptions, and successful management. He concludes that Happy Times SPCA is most likely to put his money toward more successful ventures on behalf of animals, so he writes out the check.

If Mr. Moola walked into your facility and picked up your publications, what would he think? Marketing your organization is not just about telling the public what you do and what makes you special; it's about showing them. To draw and keep donor dollars, you need to make sure that the first impressions your organization delivers are good ones.

This story about Mr. Moola's experience reinforces the point that "people are more likely to give to success"—one of the reasons listed in chapter 1 why people give.

Go through this checklist to make sure your organization looks as good as its positioning statement sounds:

■ If you operate a sheltering facility, is it welcoming? Are visitors greeted? Is the facility bright and cheerful? (Even an old building can be cheery with good staff and a fresh coat of paint.) Does it entice visitors to walk around and tour the adoption rooms, or does it cause them to run back out the door?

- Can the public find you? Is your organization listed in both the local yellow pages and white pages? If a web surfer types your organization's name into a search engine, does your name pop up? Do road signs and your building sign clearly point people in your direction?

- Have you developed strong relationships with the media to make sure your organization and its message is covered often and accurately?

- Do your newsletter, web site, and all materials designed for the public look professional and reader-friendly?

- Are the people who represent your organization competent public speakers? Are they likeable? Do they know what they are talking about?

- Does your organization mingle with the public? Do you hold community outreach events? Is your newsletter available at libraries and veterinary facilities?

People are drawn to success. To meet your fund-raising goals, your organization must not only establish its niche and package itself for the public, but it must also make sure that package looks as good on the inside as it does on the outside.

To learn more about developing effective marketing approaches for your organization, see Resources.

Chapter 3

Choosing Your Direction: How to Create a Development Plan

Here is your situation: your animal care organization needs money to help animals. Lots of people in your community have companion animals and support the concept of animal protection. Theoretically, your fund-raising strategy can consist simply of venturing out into your community with a "please help" canister, right?

Of course, it is never that simple. You know your organization does worthy work, but you cannot raise enough funds to continue that work unless you can show people what funds you already have, what funds you need, how you plan to raise more funds, and how you will manage and spend that money. How do you do this?

Get Down to Some Serious Planning

Before you can begin fund-raising for your organization, you need two plans in place, a strategic plan and a development plan. These are different tools that work together to give structure to a fund-raising program. The development plan ties directly to the strategic plan because the development plan interfaces with the organization's budgeting process.

Your organization should already be following a comprehensive, up-to-date strategic plan that charts the course for all programs, not just fund-raising. (If your organization's plan needs some fine-tuning or even a complete overhaul, see appendix B.)

With a solid strategic plan in place, complete with budget and fund-raising goals, you are ready to create your development plan, your road map for obtaining and managing funds for your animal care organization. The development planning process, like all planning processes, determines how best to achieve desired outcomes. You will find the process to be similar to your strategic planning process.

Your development plan should accomplish the following:

- Set goals to fulfill budget needs.

- Identify best and available strategies to raise funds.

- Analyze potential by constituency and strategy.

- Construct a timetable for each strategy.

- Set income and expense benchmarks for each strategy.

- Determine responsibilities for strategies and individual solicitation.

- Create a budget to fund each strategy.

- Determine marketing needs to support each strategy.

Don't Try This Alone

Your first step is to develop a consensus within your animal care organization to begin that process. You need more than an affirmative head nod from your board of directors and executive director. For the planning process to churn out a quality development plan, you need leadership's full and active support in the planning process.

The planning process involves communication and cooperation between and among all team members, staff, board members, committees, donors, and volunteers. Forming your organization's development plan should never rest on the shoulders of one person but should instead be buoyed by an entire team.

For guidance on propelling your plan from the conceptual to the concrete, consider looking outside your own organization. Outside groups like nonprofit management centers, consultants, and professional fund-raising associations can help you jump-start your plan and keep it on track. Organizations such as the Association of Fundraising Professionals are dedicated to helping nonprofit organizations manage their fund-raising programs. (For more information, see Resources.)

Starting with What You Have

When you start the development plan process, you are not starting from square one. You will be pulling information from many existing sources.

To create a development plan, you have to understand why you need to raise funds. To understand why you need money, you need to know your organization's strategic direction. That is where your organization's existing strategic plan comes in. Your development plan will incorporate your strategic plan and market research to identify strategies for fund development.

Your plan's focus must extend beyond your organization's needs to include your prospective donors' needs, too. After all, to create a workable plan, you must keep in mind the wants and perceptions of the very people the development plan targets. To do this, look at your mission statement, positioning statement, outreach materials, and other existing resources to pinpoint what your animal care organization offers to the community, whom your organization serves, what the public needs, and how you communicate with that public. (For more information on deciphering your community's needs and perceptions and communicating your distinctiveness to the public, review chapter 2.)

Although you can use many of your existing materials and your knowledge to develop your development plan, you will still have to delve into some unfamiliar territory as you dig into the planning process. You and your team will need to develop, update, and expand your organization's:

- case for support

- prospect research

- cultivation development

- solicitation strategies

- methods for acknowledging and recognizing donors

- procedures for managing gifts

Putting It All Together

Every animal care organization has different needs, so there is no one right mix of fund-raising methods and types of giving for your development plan. Still, your plan should integrate direct mail, project grants, special events, capital gifts, major gifts, and planned giving. To select fund-raising approaches to fit your needs, look at your organization's:

- need for operational income

- need for capital improvements

- need for specific programs

- prospects' level of involvement

- prospects' readiness and capacity to give

Analyzing these factors will help you project likely income, determine fund-raising strategies for your plan, and calculate the cost of those strategies to be supported by your organizational budget.

As you look at these costs, you will also need to consider how your expenditures (direct-mail campaigns and development director's salary, for example) affect your fund-raising ratio (fund-raising costs divided by total revenues). Because of a few examples of inefficient or unethical fund-raising, public scrutiny of fund-raising practices and costs has intensified. Potential donors look at figures and assume that a smaller ratio means that an organization is more efficient. In reality, an organization should be judged by more than just how much it spends on fund-raising. Don't let concerns about your ratio deter you from investing essential resources in your fund-raising program. Seek guidance from your financial advisors to evaluate and design measurement techniques and reporting formats to show contributors a fair and realistic picture of your organization's fund-raising costs and overall effectiveness.

A well-integrated development plan will provide the basic annual income to support your organization's core programs and operations; the funds needed for buildings and maintenance; and the planned gifts to provide for the future. Most organizations start with annual giving to address immediate operating needs. As your organization adds additional requirements, you will venture beyond this basic operating support to seek donations for capital needs. Make sure your plan encompasses not just your organization's immediate and short-term needs and plans but your long-term expectations as well.

Although your development plan should be comprehensive, it must also be realistic. It should strike a balance between finding funds to maintain and grow your organization and keeping approaches practical and obtainable. Your development plan doesn't have to last fifty years—you can and should update your plan as your organization progresses and its goals change.

See the following section for details and examples to help you customize a development plan that works for your animal care organization. For real-world examples, also review the forms from the Maryland SPCA provided in appendices D.1–D.4.

The Development Plan: Step-by-Step

Step 1: Set goals to fulfill budget needs.

First, identify income categories from the previous year and note actual income generated. Next, add the income projections for the upcoming year and determine the difference. Here is an example:

Table 3.1

Fund-Raising Financial Goals for the XYZ Humane Society,
Projected by Fiscal Year (FY) 2005 Operating Budget ($606,700)

Income Categories	FY 2004 Income Actual	FY 2005 Income Projected	Difference
Direct Mail	$320,000	$345,600	$25,600
Foundations	$38,000	$45,000	$7,000
Individuals/ Family Trusts	$95,200	$120,000	$24,800
Federated Campaigns (CFC, United Way)	$23,000	$25,000	$2,000
Special Events	$80,000	$90,000	$10,000
Other (Unsolicited Income)	$18,000	$5,000	-$13,000
Corporations	$30,000	$40,000	$10,000
Interest Income	$2,500	$1,800	-$700
TOTAL INCOME	**$606,700**	**$672,400**	**$65,700**

Table 3.1 shows different types of fund-raising techniques and their success over the past few years. When creating a development plan, be realistic. Getting your fund-raising operations up and running takes time.

Step 2: Identify best and available strategies.

These are non-monetary goals that will affect the success of your plan. But be realistic: until you get your fund-raising operations up and running, it is unrealistic to project significant increases in fund-raising. Here is an example:

Strategic Goals for the XYZ Humane Society

1. Achieve 100 percent giving by the XYZ Humane Society board, executive director, and key staff (92 percent giving was achieved in previous FY).

2. Achieve 100 percent participation by board in some fund-raising task, including cultivation of donors (56 percent was achieved in previous FY).

3. Enhance communications on fund development within the board and with prospects, including regular presentations at board meetings by fund development chair.

4. Develop plan for ongoing recruitment and training of fund-raising volunteers. Recruit a minimum of five non-board volunteers to work in fund development.

5. Develop new prospects for both personal solicitation campaign and direct mail solicitation. Cultivate foundations and family trusts.

6. Strengthen donor cultivation program. Improve board and staff understanding of the purpose and process of cultivation.

7. Actively involve corporate volunteers, students, board members, and staff in special events.

8. Develop coordination between public relations and fund development committees to support fund-raising efforts. Don't forget to ask for money at all opportunities.

9. Develop a process for ongoing monitoring and evaluation of progress in all areas of fund-raising.

Step 3: Analyze potential by constituency and strategy; construct a timetable and goals; set benchmarks; and assign responsibilities for each strategy.

Analyze each fund-raising method—personal solicitation, special events, direct mail, foundation grants, federated campaigns, family trusts, bequests, etc.—and spell out your strategy for each one. Here is an example:

Solicitation Strategies for the XYZ Humane Society

    A. *Personal Solicitation Campaign*

        Board Solicitation (Chairs: President, Fund Development Chair)

        Time Frame: September—December 2005

        Number of Prospects: 18

        Goal: 100 percent giving; $8,500 ($7,820 raised in previous FY)

        Method: Personal solicitation; request amounts based on giving history

        Solicitors: President and Fund Development Chair

    B. *Special Events*

        The Mighty Dog Walk (Walk Chair: Name)

        Time Frame: September 4, 2005

        Number of Walkers: 200

        Goal: $35,000 gross/$30,000 net (FY '04 walk grossed $34,000)

Table 3.2

Comparison of Reported Success of Techniques, December 2001–December 2003

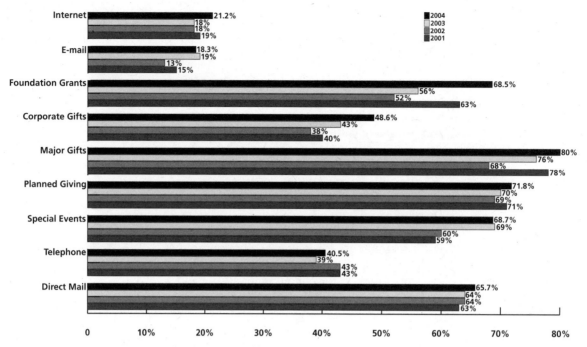

Source: The Center on Philanthropy at Indiana University 2004.

C. Method

> Mailing of 4,000 pieces; phone-a-thon two weeks later
> to recruit walkers and pledgers and to solicit donations;
> news articles and other promotional items; other
> personal recruitment by board, staff, and students

For a national comparison of reported success for different fund-raising strategies, see Table 3.2.

Step 4: Create a budget to fund each strategy.

Determine your costs for each strategy so you can reach the net goal. What can you get underwritten? What gifts-in-kind can you get? Say, for example, that at your planned dog walk you want to give each walker a T-shirt. Can you find a local T-shirt printer to donate the shirts and printing? Will the local bank agree to underwrite the T-shirts in exchange for placing its logo on the back of them? Rarely will you have extra money lying around to pay for fund-raising expenses, so incorporate into your plan what you need to have underwritten, donated, or sponsored. At the same time, realize that you will have to spend some money to make money. It doesn't make sense to spend too much staff or volunteer time going after unrealistic or unworthy "freebies."

Step 5: Determine marketing needs to support each strategy.

To develop a successful and fully integrated development plan, you will need to conduct market research to help you understand and reach out to your target market. Essentially, market research is the process of gathering, recording, and analyzing information pertaining to the marketing of goods and services. The animals you have for adoption are your goods, and your programs are your services.

Why do you need market research to complete your development plan? You need to know and understand the people likely to support and use your organization's services. Whether they are clients, donors, or volunteers, you need to learn enough about them to design your programs and approaches to fit their needs. Here is what you need to find out:

- Who are your donors?

- What are their demographic characteristics (e.g., age, gender, location, education, income)?

- Why do they give to your organization?

- What do they need and want?

- What is their lifestyle (leisure-time activities, volunteer experiences, favorite charities)?

- How do they receive information?

- Which target markets have the highest priority?

- How can you create new relationships and enhance current relationships?

- What is your niche in the community (see chapter 2)?

- What is your competition (i.e., what is unique about them, their future plans)?

- How well do you communicate with your constituents?

Taking the time to develop these data now can save you a lot of time and expense later on. The XYZ Humane Society learned this lesson the hard way. For two years it kept its adopters on its direct-mail list because the shelter wanted to turn adopters into donors. Despite all this time and expense, only 1 percent of those donors became direct-mail donors. Engaging in some market research showed the XYZ Humane Society that adoption did not necessarily translate into donation. A survey of past adopters showed that most adopters felt that they had already contributed by adopting the animals. This feedback helped the shelter change how it approached adopters. The XYZ Humane Society removed adopters from its direct-mail list (at considerable savings) and placed them instead on a "special events" and phone-a-thon list. The result? People who adopted their animals from the shelter were more likely to participate in animal-related events such as dog walks and Frisbee™ contests. These adopters also contributed to phone pledge drives for the annual telethon. By getting to know your constituents and segmenting your market, your organization, too, can create a development plan that saves time and money and brings in much-needed funds and support. Even if you are unable to conduct in-depth research, at least take time to consider your community's local economy, current socio-economic situation, and competition in the area.

Step 6: Develop cultivation strategies.

Your market research will help you tackle your next task, completing a list of your strategies for "friend-raising." Here is an example:

Cultivation Strategies for the XYZ Humane Society

The purpose of cultivation is:

1. to add prospects to the XYZ Humane Society's donor base and develop them into active supporters and regular donors

2. to improve relationships with current board members, donors, volunteers, and other friends of the XYZ Humane Society to build a greater understanding of how they can help our agency achieve its mission

Donor and volunteer recognition is critical to the cultivation process. Cultivation needs to be discussed regularly at XYZ Humane Society board meetings to encourage each board member to become part of the cultivation process.

A. *Open Houses*: Responsibility of the Public Relations Committee

Time: Twice a year: November 2005 and May 2006

Goal: Host appreciation evenings at the XYZ Humane Society for donors and volunteers; provide opportunity to see facility and meet staff; recruit potential volunteers; and cultivate potential donors

Method: Special mailings with invitations; newsletter articles; public announcements; personal invitations by the board and executive director

Responsible: board, staff, other volunteers

B. *Communications:*

Holiday Card: Holiday greeting card to four hundred friends and major donors

Newsletter: Published four times a year and sent to our mailing list; provides regular updates on programs, activities, and special events

Annual Report: Annual report to coincide with the fiscal year (September 1); mailing in November a major communications tool sent to funding sources, major donors, agency executives, public officials, and media contacts; submitted with most proposals and requests to major donor prospects

C. *Other P.R.:*

A separate public relations plan to be developed by the Public Relations Committee to help reinforce cultivation efforts of the fund development plan; the Fund Development Committee and Public Relations Committee must maintain close communication to adequately support the objectives of the fund development plan

Table 3.3

Percentage of Donors Who Were New to U.S. Charities in 2003

What percentage of your donors were new in 2003?	Percentage of U.S. Charities
1–5	28.8
6–10	30.9
11–15	17.7
16–20	9.4
21–25	4.0
26+	9.1

Source: Association of Fundraising Professionals 2004.

Table 3.4

Percentage of Continuing Donors Who Increased Their Gift to U.S. Charities in 2003

Percentage of Continuing Donors Who Increased Their Gift to U.S. Charities in 2003	Percentage of U.S. Charities
1–5	36.2
6–10	30.9
11–15	15.0
16–20	6.4
21–25	4.7
26+	6.7

Source: Association of Fundraising Professionals 2004.

Keep in mind that different methods of cultivation should be used for different segments of your donor file. Donors at different levels are more likely to respond to specific cultivation tools. For example, in direct-mail solicitation, higher-end donors are more likely to respond to personalized appeals in closed-face envelopes. (For data on new donors and existing supporters, see tables 3.3 and 3.4.) Keep in mind that while new-donor dollars help, the majority of your funds will come from repeat donors who may not give more but who give consistently.

Step 7: Determine how to monitor your development plan.

Here is an example:

Monitoring the XYZ Humane Society Fund Development Plan and Process

1. The Fund Development Committee will meet eight times a year to review the progress of the plan and, with fund development staff, will identify problems and solutions.

2. Development staff and committee chair will discuss issues regularly.

3. Development chair will report the progress at regular board meetings.

4. Development staff will provide financial and statistical data to help evaluate the plan's progress.

Step 8: Create yearly fund development calendar.

This is the last step in writing your development plan. Here is an example:

XYZ Humane Society Fund Development Calendar, FY 2005

September	Prepare Annual Report Review results of August telethon
October	Prepare holiday mailing lists P.R. Committee plans open house Personal Campaign with major donors Direct mail #2 planned

Chapter 4

Following the Rules:
How to Meet Legal Requirements
and Ethical Expectations

Newlyweds are often told, "If you don't have trust, you don't have anything." This is true for your organization, too. Public trust is the most important asset of your animal care organization. Without it, donors will not give and volunteers will not get involved.

The rights and privileges granted to your organization and other nonprofits stem from the trust placed in you to promote the public good. Recently, however, a few prominent nonprofit and for-profit organizations have engaged in unethical and illegal activities, such as deceptive accounting, that have eroded that trust. Their actions, made public by the media, are making your job more difficult.

No longer can nonprofits simply be do-gooders. Nonprofits must act ethically and be held accountable for achieving results. Your animal care organization's ability to raise the funds necessary to help your community depends on your organization's ability to gain the public's confidence. To do that, you not only have to do good, you have to be good—and prove it.

Legal and ethical issues will arise that tie directly and indirectly to your money-raising practices. This chapter provides an overview and some direction on these issues but cannot provide a complete, comprehensive guide on all legal and ethical considerations. To learn more, consult your attorney and see Resources.

Who Is Responsible?

The ethical and legal behavior of your animal care organization is the ultimate responsibility of its board of directors. As lawful owner and ethical steward of your organization, the board of directors is the first line of defense against misuse of charitable dollars. This is a hefty responsibility for the board members. If your organization's board is committed to animals but not to financial and legal oversight, your organization is in jeopardy. Board members who do not understand the financial aspects of an organization are a huge liability, not just to the organization, but to themselves as well. Many board members rise from volunteer ranks, attaining their positions through "sweat equity" but lacking basic information on finances. Make sure all board members receive sufficient training to fulfill their duties (see chapter 5 and appendix C for ways to accomplish this).

Your staff and volunteers may not be charged with this overarching responsibility, but they should be charged with carrying out their duties responsibly. Their daily routines, however basic, can still affect the legal, financial, and ethical health of your organization. For example, what happens if an eager, self-motivated volunteer initiates a well-intentioned but poorly planned fund-raiser in your name and without your knowledge? Make sure your staff and volunteers understand that they must get authorization for any fund-raising activity. Along with the standard policies and procedures that you provide all staff and volunteers, be sure to include your organization's fund-raising policies. For more information about the role of boards, staff, and volunteers, see chapter 5 and appendix C.

A Bit of Law School

Ethical behavior and accountability begin with compliance with all applicable local, state, and federal laws and regulations. Government has a key role to play in enforcing minimum standards of practice for all charities, but any high-functioning animal care organization will reach beyond those minimum requirements.

Meeting even the minimum requirements takes preparation and follow-through. Here's a breakdown of the basic federal and state laws you will need to know:

Be a 501(c)(3)

This manual is written for those nonprofit animal care organizations that have incorporated in their state and been recognized as 501(c)(3) organizations by the Internal Revenue Service (IRS). It is not enough to behave like a nonprofit organization and begin accepting donations, nor is it automatic that your group is exempt from taxation. It is not ethical to let donors assume that their gifts are tax-deductible if you have not applied for and obtained this official recognition from the IRS.

For detailed information on becoming a documented charity, speak to your accountant or lawyer and read *How to Form a Humane Organization*, published by The HSUS. The IRS also has excellent publications available at *www.irs.gov*. Publication 4220, *Applying for 501(c)(3) Tax-Exempt Status*, is designed to help prospective charities apply for tax exemption.

Return Those Returns

Your animal care organization must keep books and records to show that it complies with tax regulations. It must be able to document the sources of receipts and expenditures on IRS Form 990, *Return of Organization Exempt from Income Tax*. Form 990 must be filed annually with the IRS by organizations with $25,000 or more in income.

Form 990 is becoming increasingly complex for nonprofits to complete. Total operating expenses must be accounted for in three separate groupings: program services, management and general, and fund-raising. The IRS has also intensified its oversight of nonprofit fund-raising activities, so it is even more critical that your organization make sure that all fund-raising costs are segregated, reported, and allocated properly. If you are not careful, your organization could incur substantial penalties. That is why it's important to work with a tax professional—one not on the board or associated with your organization—who can advise you on the level of detail that must be maintained to complete your income tax returns and financial statements.

Who Wants to Know?

Your animal care organization does not have to submit to public elections, nor do your "customers" determine bottom line of profit or loss. So to help make nonprofit organizations more accountable to the public that funds them, the IRS requires that certain documents be made publicly available. The disclosure law requires that you produce:

1. Form 990 or 990-EZ. The three most recent returns must be made available, along with any filed attachments. (Make sure you mask the names and addresses of contributors on copies released to the public.) You are also required to disclose the amounts of contributions and bequests, unless sharing that information would identify contributors.

2. Form 1023. A charitable organization's application for exemption (Form 1023), any attachments to the application, and any materials the IRS requests in connection with the application must be disclosed.

3. Letter of determination. The public is entitled to see your organization's IRS letter of determination that stipulates that it is a charitable organization.

If someone comes into your office to request this information, you usually need to fulfill the request that day. If you receive the request in writing, you have thirty days to comply. Your organization can charge the requester "reasonable copying costs" for the document in question. (The IRS allows one dollar for the first page and fifteen cents for each subsequent page.)

What happens if you do not comply with the request? The penalty for not disclosing an annual return is twenty dollars per day until you comply, up to $10,000 per return not disclosed. There is no maximum fee for failure to provide the application for exemption.

You can bypass the hard copy hassle by posting copies of these documents on your organization's web site. Like the hard copies, the documents shown on your web site cannot be altered, except to mask donors' names and contact information. Consider making your annual return and even optional information (such as your mission, goals, staff, and board of directors) available on GuideStar, a national database of nonprofit organizations, and refer those requesting information to *www.guidestar.org*. In fact, your animal care organization's information may already be on that web site; GuideStar obtains the documents directly from the IRS and posts them to its web site.

More information about disclosure regulations is available on the IRS web site (*www.irs.gov*) and in Resources.

Be a Good Boss

Employment laws may seem far removed from fund-raising, but following them certainly affects your organization's ability to maintain its donor base. That is because few things will undermine an organization's reputation in the community or the loyalty of its employees faster than failing to pay all appropriate employment taxes on time or failing to follow overtime provisions of the Labor Code. Ethical and legal responsibility begins with an organization's role as an honest employer. See Resources for a list of helpful resources.

Gifts with Strings

The most basic rule of fund-raising is that the donors must actually give away funds. They cannot receive goods and services in return for their gifts, nor can they obtain dividends on their investment. Donors can receive recognition and small tokens of appreciation, but if they receive a monetary return for the donation, they will lose their tax deduction, and the nonprofit organization could lose its tax exemption.

Under the Omnibus Budget Reconciliation Act of 1993, the IRS requires "specific substantiation"—proof—of tax-deductible donations to charity. While other legal requirements for nonprofits are best left to accountants and lawyers, the standard for gift substantiation will be used daily by your animal care organization's fund-raising staff.

Adhering to these two general rules will help you meet substantiation and disclosure requirements for federal income tax return reporting purposes:

1. A donor must obtain a written acknowledgment from a charity for any single contribution of $250 or more before the donor can claim a charitable contribution on his federal income tax return.

2. A charitable organization must provide a written disclosure to a donor who makes a payment in excess of $75 that is partly a donation and partly for goods and services provided by the organization.

To be deductible, a payment to a qualified charitable organization must be a gift. No meal, gift, service, or value can be received in return for a contribution. If there is, the organization must provide a "good faith" estimate of the value of the goods or services, and the donor must reduce the amount of the deduction by the fair market value of the goods and services provided. All this can be confusing to charities and donors and result in reporting errors on both sides. Consequently, the IRS now monitors these exchanges more closely.

One special category of donation is the "gift-in-kind." Gifts-in-kind include most non-cash personal property donations (such as automobiles, works of art, furniture, and equipment) and gifts of services (such as photography, veterinary, legal, or accounting services). Gifts-in-kind require special processing to ensure that tax regulations are satisfied and that the gift is recorded properly in the organization's financial statements. While the nonprofit will provide a letter of acknowledgment for the gift-in-kind donation, it does not assign a value to the donation. For tax receipt purposes, it is the responsibility of the donor to substantiate to the IRS the value of the gift. When a gift of personal property is valued at $5,000 or more, the IRS requires an independent appraisal. Keep in mind that while in-kind gifts can be great if the organization can use them, some "gifts of property" can be more trouble than they are worth. People who donate their property (jewelry or an old car, for example) may be motivated by favorable tax deduction rules, leaving the organization to net far less than the value of the claimed deduction. If you accept property, consider how you will safeguard the gift or sell it. Find out whether you will acquire liability risks when you acquire the property. For example, what if the donated building burns down before you can sell it? Who was responsible for the fire insurance policy? What if someone is seriously injured on the property, say, by falling in the swimming pool? When in doubt about whether and how to accept a gift, get advice from a professional.

To better understand the substantiation and disclosure requirements for the gifts you do accept, take a look at these basic examples:

Example 1. Ms. Cat Lover writes a $500 check to the XYZ Humane Society to sterilize cats. Because the gift is over $250, the donor will need a written acknowledgment. Because there was no gift or service to the donor, the acknowledgment will state that the full $500 is deductible for IRS purposes.

Example 2. Ms. Dog Lover writes a check for $100 to the XYZ Humane Society in response to its annual appeal for donations. The Humane Society is not required to provide any written acknowledgment because the gift was under $250 and no goods or services were provided. But the organization better make sure it sends a thank-you note to Ms. Dog Lover for supporting its work!

Example 3. Ms. Cat Lover purchases four tickets to the XYZ Humane Society's annual black-tie gala. The tickets cost $125 each and a check totaling $500 is written to the humane society. In this case the donor is receiving a benefit (dinner and dancing) with a fair market value of $75 per ticket. The organization's written disclosure must state that the donor received a benefit of $75 per ticket, for a total of $300, and that only $200 is allowed as a deduction for IRS purposes. The donor made a gift partly as a contribution and partly for goods and services provided by XYZ Humane Society. This contribution is known as a quid pro quo contribution.

Example 4. During a benefit auction at the XYZ Humane Society's black-tie gala dinner-dance, Ms. Cat Lover wins a popular diamond-studded cat collar with her bid of $1,000. She then writes a $1,000 check to XYZ Humane Society for the collar, which has a fair market value of $750. This transaction is a quid pro quo donation—Ms. Cat Lover received a $750 cat collar in exchange for her $1,000 "contribution." She can deduct only the amount ($250) that she paid above the collar's value as a donation, and the XYZ Humane Society must provide her with a written disclosure to substantiate this.

Example 5. During a benefit auction at the XYZ Humane Society black tie gala, Ms. Dog Lover wins a sapphire-studded dog collar with her bid of $500. The fair market value of the collar is $750, exceeding by $250 the amount she pays to XYZ Humane Society. So when the XYZ Humane Society sends her a written disclosure for her $500 purchase, it must state that goods and services with a value of $750 were received for the $500 payment and none of Ms. Dog Lover's purchase price for the collar will be deductible for tax purposes.

Example 6. Ms. Cat Lover's husband is an accountant who donated a gift for the silent auction at XYZ Humane Society's black-tie gala. His gift—two hours of his accounting expertise—sells for $300 at the party. The value of one's time or services is not deductible as a charitable contribution. Although Mr. Cat Lover will receive a nice thank-you note from the organization, he will not receive any receipt for his gift.

Example 7. Ms. Dog Lover's husband owns a nursery and donates a gift for the XYZ Humane Society's benefit auction: a $400 tree and $200 worth of labor to plant the tree. He is able to deduct the fair market value of his gift of property (the tree) but is not able to deduct the labor (a gift of service). The XYZ Humane Society must state this clearly in the receipt it gives him.

Since not every gift to a nonprofit organization is deductible, you must keep your eyes open for inappropriate gift claims. Scrutinize the receipts you provide donors to make sure they are clear and valid. Your organization does not want to hear from angry donors who are told by the IRS that they claimed an invalid gift amount. Truthful advertising of events and substantiation of contributions is a fundamental requirement for any nonprofit.

Keeping track of all of the complicated requirements for written disclosure and written acknowledgment for contributions is not easy. See Resources for other sources for guidance on complying with these rules.

True or False?

■ If your animal care organization uses the full amount of a donor's contribution for charitable purposes, then that donor can deduct that full amount even if she received something in return.

> **Answer:** False. If the donor received basic goods or services for her donation, it is still a quid pro quo contribution, and the donor can deduct only the amount above the fair market value of what she received.

■ If a donor ends up not using the tickets he bought to attend your animal care organization's black-tie gala fund-raising event, then the full amount the donor paid is tax deductible.

Answer: False. The fact that tickets or other privileges were not used does not change the fact that those goods or services were provided. For tax purposes, the donor must still subtract the fair market value of those tickets from the amount he gave to your organization.

■ The cost of raffle tickets is not tax-deductible.

Answer: True. Charities should be careful to avoid any wording that implies that raffle tickets are a deductible gift.

Before You Start That Business

Your tax-exempt organization is not taxed on money it makes through activities substantially related to its charitable purposes. However, if your animal care organization regularly carries on a trade or business that is not substantially related to its charitable purposes, then the organization must pay taxes on that income. This is called Unrelated Business Income Tax.

Determining whether that income is "substantially related" entails more than just guesswork. According to the IRS, determining if a business activity is substantially related requires

> [E]xamining the relationship between the activities that generate income and the accomplishment of the organization's exempt purpose....The activities that generate income must contribute importantly to accomplishing the organization's exempt purposes to be substantially related. (Internal Revenue Service, n.d., n.p.)

IRS Publication 598, *Tax on Unrelated Business Income of Exempt Organizations*, specifically addresses animal care organizations on this issue. An organization operated for the prevention of cruelty to animals that offers pet boarding and grooming services for the general public receives unrelated business income from these services. The IRS would therefore tax the gross income from the boarding and grooming, less the deductions to carry out this business. If the gross income is $1,000 or more, Form 990-T must be filed and any required taxes must be paid.

Here volunteers can make all the difference. If uncompensated volunteers perform all the work in your animal care organization's trade or business, it is not considered an unrelated business. Also, if the business consists of selling merchandise donated to your organization, this, too, is not considered unrelated business income. (It is no wonder why so many nonprofit organizations operate thrift shops run by volunteers!)

If your animal care organization plans to conduct activities or business ventures to augment its income, do not take chances with complicated tax laws. Make sure you run everything by a tax professional.

It's Not Just the Fed

Most states have adopted charitable solicitation laws designed to protect donors, the general public, and charities themselves from fraud. Generally, these laws require charities and their outside, hired fund-raisers to register with the state, describe their fund-raising activities, file financial documents, and pay a fee that covers the administrative expenses of monitoring charities.

If this leaves you scratching your head, you are not alone; state registration is probably the most common fund-raising requirement overlooked by nonprofits. While the IRS governs tax breaks for the organization and donors, state governments are the most active regulators of fund-raising.

If you raise funds in a state without first registering, you may be risking hefty fines. Visit *www.multistatefiling.org* for registration information and forms for states requiring registration.

The registration rules are relatively straightforward, except when it comes to fund-raising over the Internet. (Learn more about online fund-raising in chapter 12.)

No One Likes a Fraud

State registration is no guarantee that contributions reach the nonprofit or help a good cause. Sometimes organizations spend more on fund-raising than they receive. Because fund-raising appeals are considered protected free speech, states cannot mandate that a certain percentage of the funds raised go to the organization's charitable activities. States can insist, however, that the charity or its fund-raiser tell the truth when soliciting funds. Diligent donors ask careful questions, and it is your organization's ethical and legal duty to answer these questions truthfully.

The Federal Trade Commission recently launched "Operation Phoney Philanthropy," a law enforcement and public education campaign designed to help donors recognize and avoid bogus charities and fraudulent fund-raising. The campaign urges donors to verify a charity's legitimacy. Donors can find this information at *www.ftc.gov/charityfraud*.

You probably have heard about new national requirements that telemarketers abide by a national "do not call" registry. Although your animal care organization and other charities are exempt from this requirement, you should still honor all "do not call" requests from individuals.

As this new national do-not-call list begins to dry up business for commercial telemarketers, they may start calling on your organization. Be wary of their too-good-to-be-true offers to raise money on your behalf. The amount your organization receives may be no more than 10 percent of all the money raised. Your donors rightfully expect their generous contributions to be used to help animals, not to enrich telemarketing firms. Partnering with telemarketing and direct-mail firms can pose some ethical quandaries. How much of a donor's dollar should go to pay the private contractor? Is it ethical to raise $100,000 if $90,000 goes to the private contractor doing the work? What if the organization needs that $10,000 and could not have raised it without the help of the contractor? What if the breakdown is 80–20 or 50–50? Before teaming up with a telemarketing firm, analyze whether the partnership is in the best interest of your organization, its reputation, and its donors.

Adding It All Up

Fund-raising brings a very obvious benefit—money—but it also makes your record-keeping system more complex. Although the law does not require a special kind of record or system, it is critical that your system creates clear income and expense reports and maintains accurate records of all donations, other income, and all expenses.

What happens if your records consist of a few yellowed scraps of paper with illegible scribbles? If your organization cannot produce complete and accurate financial records, your board cannot govern the organization, and your organization cannot demonstrate its qualification for tax exemption, it cannot fill out its tax returns, and it may be subject to penalties.

Good records don't just keep your organization out of trouble, they can also help pinpoint which programs are succeeding and which are in danger of failing. In an era of savvy donors and funders, it is no longer enough to say, "We adopted out 117 cats"; you also must show that your organization accomplished this in a financially reasonable way and that it used contributions responsibly.

You will also find that maintaining good financial records now will help you deal with the IRS later. For example, you will feel much less frustrated over the IRS's intricate requirements for recording gifts if you have a system for tracking donations, end-of-the-year gifts, non-cash gifts, hard credits/soft credits, and other complex classifications. If these terms do not sound familiar, you may not be the one to manage your financial record system. Have someone experienced in finances, taxes, and legal requirements develop this system for your organization.

The person responsible for your accounting and taxes should use Generally Accepted Accounting Principles (GAAP), which provide minimum standards, guidelines, and policy for financial accounting and reporting. The central theme of GAAP is accountability. GAAP ensures that a reader of financial information will be reviewing financial data and reports that are consistent, comparable, and present fairly the financial results of an organization. GAAP varies by the type of organization. Most animal care organizations will fall under the GAAP requirements for a municipal government or private nonprofit organization. Because financial statements of different animal care organizations are reported in a similar way, donors can compare "apples to apples" when analyzing organizations' financial situations.

Another term often used in connection with financial reporting is "FASB requirements"—rules promulgated by the Financial Accounting Standards Board. Since 1995 the Financial Accounting Standards Board Statement Number 117 has required that nonprofit organizations produce:

■ a Statement of Financial Position (Balance Sheet)

■ a Statement of Activities (Income Statement)

■ a Statement of Cash Flows

■ a Statement of Functional Expenses (required for some organizations, but useful for all nonprofits)

■ Notes (Footnotes)

When your board and other reviewers examine these financial records, three key figures should stand out:

1. percentage spent on fund-raising and management

2. total assets

3. cost of salaries

Standards put out by the Institute of Philanthropy Standards and the Combined Federal Campaign serve as guidelines on how much money nonprofit organizations should spend on program activities, fund-raising, and management expenses:

■ At least 60 percent of the annual budget should be spent on program activities.

■ Fund-raising and management expenses should not exceed 25 percent of the annual budget. (In the animal care and control field, salaries and wages typically are 50 percent or more of the organization's annual budget.)

These general guidelines can provide quick indicators of the organization's basic performance. If the percentages in your organization's report fall outside these ranges, it is time to do some fact checking. Either the financial statements do not state the organization's activities accurately or your organization's practices deviate from the norm. Neither the IRS nor any other federal agency requires audited financial statements, but state charitable registrars, banks, and many foundations often ask for them.

Obey More than the Law

Many people tend to follow the law, not out of moral obligation but out of fear of reprisal. Many organizations follow federal and state requirements, not because they should, but because they want to avoid financial penalties. Of course, some people and organizations skirt these laws anyway, despite risk of punishment, so it is no surprise that it can be challenging to get people and organizations to abide by ethics—the principles of conduct governing an individual or a group. Why should you fret about extra ethical duties when legal requirements already demand so much effort? Because it is the right thing to do, and nonprofits are all about doing the right thing, not just for the animals or schools or churches they serve but also for the greater community.

Your donors know this. They expect that the do-gooders they support do good and are good. If your organization fails, it will fail to draw in the dollars and community backing necessary to survive. In fact, even if your organization has a reasonable explanation to counter an accusation of impropriety, the mere perception of unethical conduct can cause irreparable harm.

Here are some of your ethical duties tied to fund-raising.

Conflict of Interest

While state laws governing nonprofit corporations usually set the legal definition of conflict of interest, most conflicts fall into a gray area where ethics and public perception are more relevant than statutes.

Conflicts of interest are common in nonprofit charities. A board member, for example, wears many hats and has many community contacts. Is it a conflict of interest if the board member provides professional services for the organization or recommends that a friend be considered for a staff position? Such transactions are perfectly acceptable if they benefit the organization and receive approval from an objective and informed board. Even if they do not meet these standards, such transactions are usually not illegal. They are, however, vulnerable to legal challenges and public misunderstanding. Loss of public confidence and a damaged reputation are the most likely results of a poorly managed conflict-of-interest policy. Because public confidence is so important, boards should take steps to avoid even the appearance of impropriety. The board should never lose sight of its basic obligations: duty of care, duty of loyalty, and duty of obedience.

BoardSource, a resource for many board-of-directors issues (*www.boardsource.org/FullAnswer.asp?ID=89*), offers these recommendations:

■ Adopt a conflict-of-interest policy that prohibits or limits business transactions with board members and requires board members to disclose potential conflicts.

■ Disclose conflicts when they occur so that board members voting on a decision are aware that another member's interests are being affected.

■ Require board members to withdraw from decisions that present a potential conflict.

■ Establish procedures, such as competitive bids, to ensure that the organization is receiving fair value in the transaction.

Protecting the broad public good and upholding ethical behavior is the responsibility of every board member, but many organizations have every staff member and volunteer sign a conflict-of-interest statement, too.

See appendix D.5 for a sample conflict-of-interest policy.

Not All Gifts or Givers Are Acceptable

The Maryland Nonprofits Standards for Excellence Program recommends that you refrain from automatically accepting all gifts from all donors. Develop policies that spell out which gifts or donors are not acceptable. For example, before taking a gift from, say, a prosperous farmer who sells purebred puppies to pet stores, first consider whether accepting that contribution could jeopardize the reputation of your organization or undermine its efforts in any way. Different organizations may come to different conclusions. For example, some organizations may view accepting such a gift as counter to their mission and values. Conversely, other organizations may conclude that accepting the gift is ethically justifiable in that it allows the organization to help more animals and reach out to educate the farmer. Creating ironclad rules can be difficult. Do you accept donations from a pet store that sells rodents and reptiles but that also provides off-site adoption opportunities for your organization? Would you accept money from someone who sells turtles or fish or birds?

Before reaching for any gift, ask yourself these questions:

- Is the gift relevant to the work and mission of the organization?

- Will accepting the gift jeopardize the reputation of the donor or the organization? Does the donor's intent match the interests of the organization?

- Will the gift cost the organization money in the future, such as maintenance, repair, or preservation costs?

- Are there any risks associated with accepting the gift?

- Will the gift require a special facility in which to house it?

- Is the donor imposing any special conditions?

- If the property cannot be used in the organization's programs, will the donor allow it to be sold? If not, should the organization accept the gift?

Just as you are smart to ask questions before accepting donations, most donors are smart to ask questions before donating to your organization. These may include:

- Does the organization do what it says it does?

- Does it do it efficiently and ethically?

- Is what it does effective in solving the problem?

- Is this the best organization to achieve the results desired from my philanthropic investment?

- Is the organization growing? If so, is it growing to meet community needs?

- Is the problem an important one in the community, and are other organizations working on the same problem?

- Does the organization describe its customers in respectful ways?

- Does it acknowledge its funders and supporters?

- Does it measure program outcomes?
  If so, are the outcomes acceptable?

- Does it have a stable board and staff?

- Does it use and honor volunteers?

These donor inquiries go beyond the ethical practices of your organization. Donors expect your organization to be well governed, managed, and organized. If it isn't, it won't get many donor dollars, and it cannot fulfill its promise to the public and obligation to the animals.

Log onto *www.standardsforexcellence.org* and review Resources for help in developing standards in ethical practices and accountability for all aspects of your organization: mission and program; governing body; conflicts of interest; human resources; financial and legal; openness; fund-raising; and public affairs and public policy.

Respecting Donor Rights

Fund-raising is a donor-centered activity. It is all about engaging and cultivating donors so you can help them meet their philanthropic goals. This process elicits highly personal, confidential information from prospective donors. Protecting donor privacy and confidential information is a legal and ethical requirement and essential to maintaining the public's trust.

The Donor Bill of Rights provides a solid foundation and guidance for how nonprofit organizations should treat all donors:

Donor Bill of Rights

Philanthropy is based on voluntary action for the common good. It is a tradition of giving and sharing that is primary to the quality of life. To ensure that philanthropy merits the respect and trust of the general public, and that donors and prospective donors can have full confidence in the nonprofit organizations and causes they are asked to support, we declare that all donors have these rights:

I. To be informed of the organization's mission, of the way the organization intends to use donated resources, and of its capacity to use donations effectively for their intended purposes.

II. To be informed of the identity of those serving on the organization's governing board, and to expect the board to exercise prudent judgment in its stewardship responsibilities.

III. To have access to the organization's most recent financial statements.

IV. To be assured their gifts will be used for the purposes for which they were given.

V. To receive appropriate acknowledgment and recognition.

VI. To be assured that information about their donation
is handled with respect and with confidentiality to
the extent provided by law.

VII. To expect that all relationships with individuals
representing organizations of interest to the
donor will be professional in nature.

VIII. To be informed whether those seeking
donations are volunteers, employees of
the organization, or hired solicitors.

IX. To have the opportunity for their names
to be deleted from mailing lists that an
organization may intend to share.

X. To feel free to ask questions when making a donation
and to receive prompt, truthful, and forthright answers.

*(The American Association of Fund Raising Counsel, Association
for Healthcare Philanthropy, Association of Fundraising Professionals,
and the Council for Advancement and Support of Education n.d.)*

Online fund-raising adds another layer of complexity to donor relations; see chapter 12
for the "e-donor bill of rights."

Respecting Other Organizations

Ethical fund-raising demands that you treat other organizations respectfully even if you do not
agree with their policies. Do not try to win support for your organization by criticizing the work
of other animal care organizations.

For example, a limited-admission (often called "no kill") shelter should never publicly condemn
the role of open-admission shelters that must euthanize some animals to alleviate suffering, disease,
and overcrowding. Unfortunately, such bad-mouthing is commonly seen in direct mail appeals.
It is fine to share openly what your organization believes and does, but in so doing, do not make
unfavorable comparisons and judgments about other organizations' approaches.

Instead, find ways to compliment other responsible animal care organizations while drawing
attention to the special role your organization plays in the community. Supporters will view your
organization as strong and confident and will appreciate how the animal care community works
together to help animals. (For suggestions on avoiding divisive language, see chapter 7.)

A Model Code of Ethics

Following a trend in fund-raising, responsible nonprofits now adhere to a set of ethical
standards that are more stringent than those required by law.

The Association of Fundraising Professionals (AFP) (n.d.) has developed Standards
of Professional Practice for its fund-raising members:

Professional obligations:

- Members shall not engage in activities that harm the members' organization, clients, or profession.

- Members shall not engage in activities that conflict with their fiduciary, ethical, and legal obligations to their organizations and their clients.

- Members shall effectively disclose all potential and actual conflicts of interest; such disclosure does not preclude or imply ethical impropriety.

- Members shall not exploit any relationship with a donor, prospect, volunteer, or employee to the benefit of the members or the members' organizations.

- Members shall comply with all applicable local, state, provincial, and federal, civil, and criminal laws.

- Members recognize their individual boundaries of competence and are forthcoming and truthful about their professional experience and qualifications.

Solicitation and use of philanthropic funds:

- Members shall take care to ensure that all solicitation materials are accurate and correctly reflect their organization's mission and use of solicited funds.

- Members shall take care to ensure that donors receive informed, accurate, and ethical advice about the value and tax implications of contributions.

- Members shall take care to ensure that contributions are used in accordance with donors' intentions.

- Members shall take care to ensure proper stewardship of charitable contributions, including timely reports on the use and management of funds.

- Members shall obtain explicit consent by the donor before altering the conditions of a gift.

Presentation of information:

- Members shall not disclose privileged or confidential information to unauthorized parties.

- Members shall adhere to the principle that all donor and prospect information created by, or on behalf of, an organization is the property of that organization and shall not be transferred or utilized except on behalf of that organization.

- Members shall give donors the opportunity to have their names removed from lists that are sold to, rented to, or exchanged with other organizations.

- Members shall, when stating fund-raising results, use accurate and consistent accounting methods that conform to the appropriate guidelines adopted by the American Institute of Certified Public Accountants (AICPA) for the type of organization involved.

Compensation:

- Members shall not accept compensation that is based on a percentage of contributions; nor shall they accept finder's fees.

- Members may accept performance-based compensation, such as bonuses, provided such bonuses are in accord with prevailing practices within the members' own organizations, and are not based on a percentage of charitable contributions.

- Members shall not pay finder's fees, commissions, or percentage compensation based on charitable contributions and shall take care to discourage their organizations from making such payments.

The AFP has also developed the Code of Ethical Principles and Standards of Professional Practice. Everyone in your organization should follow these ethical standards:

- Practice their profession with integrity, honesty, truthfulness, and adherence to the absolute obligation to safeguard the public trust.

- Act according to the highest standards and visions of their organization, profession, and conscience.

- Put philanthropic mission above personal gain.

- Inspire others through their own sense of dedication and high purpose.

- Improve their professional knowledge and skills, so that their performance will better serve others.

- Demonstrate concern for the interests and well-being of individuals affected by their actions.

- Value the privacy, freedom of choice, and interests of all those affected by their actions.

- Foster cultural diversity and pluralistic values and treat all people with dignity and respect.

- Affirm, through personal giving, a commitment to philanthropy and its role in society.

- Adhere to the spirit as well as the letter of all applicable laws and regulations.

- Advocate within their organizations adherence to all applicable laws and regulations.

- Avoid even the appearance of any criminal offense or professional misconduct.

- Bring credit to the fund-raising profession by their public demeanor.

- Encourage colleagues to embrace and practice these ethical principles and standards of professional practice.

- Be aware of the codes of ethics promulgated by other professional organizations that serve philanthropy.

Self-regulation, as outlined by the AFP, should become common practice for all animal care organizations.

Raising Funds Right

Marilyn Fischer (2000, 21) outlines three basic value commitments for fund-raisers:

- Commitment to the organizational mission that directs the work

- Commitment to our professional relationships with the people with whom we interact

- Commitment to our own sense of personal integrity

Fischer stresses the importance of independent judgment, moral courage, and responsibility for those involved in fund-raising. Many of those new to fund-raising are also new to the fact that raising money comes with strings attached, involves tough decisions, and raises ethical dilemmas. Everyone agrees that money needs to be raised, but disagreements often arise over what to do and what is "right."

Ethical practice is complex. It is not only the black-and-white legalities that challenge fund-raisers but also the grayer ethical decisions they face. You must continually review what's right for the organizational mission, relationships with donors, and personal integrity. As you struggle with these tough choices, review the impact of each of these three specific areas to help you make the best decision.

It is impossible to anticipate every ethical situation that your organization will face in fund-raising. That is why every fund-raiser must engage in self-evaluation, and every organization must submit to a regular ethics audit that entails critical examination of your organization's ethics-related practices, policies, and procedures. An "ethics audit" is a broad term that can be categorized further into different types of audits—compliance audits, cultural audits, and systems audits. To learn more about ethics audits and determining which type fits your organization's objectives, visit *www.ethics.org*.

The Independent Sector (*www.independentsector.org*) strongly recommends that all nonprofits develop a statement of values and a code of ethics to help guide their policies, decision making, and operations. Before committing to a fund-raising proposal, decision makers should consider several questions. What is right rather than expedient? What is good rather than simply practical? What acts must never be engaged in or condoned?

Plenty of resources exist to help your organization follow the law and develop ethical standards. But just as every organization is different, every organization will vary in how it selects and applies these standards. The long-term credibility and viability of your animal care organization require that it do this diligently.

Chapter 5

Deciding Who Does What: How to Involve Your Board, Staff, and Volunteers in Fund-Raising

It's "pop quiz" time: Who in your organization should be involved in fund-raising:

        A. Your board

        B. Your staff

        C. Your volunteers

        D. All of the above

It is likely that you have taken enough multiple-choice quizzes in your life to have selected the correct answer: "D. All the above." But for most animal care organizations, putting that correct answer into practice poses a much greater challenge.

Everyone in your organization is a fund-raiser, from the staff at the front desk to the officer in the field, from the veterinary technician to the executive director, from the directors to the volunteers. Many people do not realize that, by simply sharing the passion they have for your organization with everyone they know and meet, they are beginning the process of raising money. How all these representatives interact with others will create your organization's standing in its community.

But what answer would you choose if you were given this question instead: Who in your organization is responsible for ensuring that your organization raises the funds necessary to carry out its programs and services? If you selected, "A. Your board," then you are two-for-two. As the legal corporate entity of your animal care organization, your board of directors is legally and morally accountable to the community. Among its many responsibilities is ensuring the fiscal integrity and financial health of your organization. Bluntly put, if your board is not involved in contributing and raising funds for your organization, then your board is not fulfilling its legal and ethical responsibilities.

Unfortunately, that truth alone typically is not enough to get most boards moving. If, for example, your board is falling apart from infighting, apathy, or micromanagement, board participation in fund-raising is the least of your organization's worries. Solving these underlying problems must be tackled before you can expect to make much progress getting board members to help with fund-raising. For help with board basics, see appendix C.

Of course, even a strong board—one that sees the big picture, communicates openly, conducts itself professionally, and plays well with others—often needs some prodding to go prospecting. To get your animal care organization's board members involved in fund-raising, you must first engage them in your mission—that is where motivation starts.

Empowering Your Board

Before criticizing your board for its lack of involvement, make sure that you are involving your board.

The title "board member" does not automatically turn a person into an expert or eager fund-raiser. You need to find ways to educate, empower, and motivate your board members so they can fulfill their fund-raising responsibilities.

This responsibility starts with the nominating committee, which must fully disclose to candidates all roles and responsibilities (especially as they relate to personal contributions and fund-raising) during the recruiting process. Don't wait until a new member has been elected to the board to start the process.

The steps below can help you empower your board to fund-raise. (Many of these steps can be replicated for your staff and volunteers, too.)

- **Provide a crash course.** Require that all new board members attend a formal orientation session that exposes them to your organization's purpose, mission, philosophy, services, and goals. If your board members cannot tell potential donors effectively what your organization is, what it does, and why money is important to help you fulfill your mission and goals, then they cannot be successful fund-raisers.

- **Involve members.** Make sure to include your board in any planning process designed to determine what the organization wants and what it will do. You want your board to feel and be a part of your organization's goals, objectives, programs, and services.

- **Stress basic responsibilities.** Before bringing on a new board member, be up-front about all legal and ethical board responsibilities as well as the ramifications of not fulfilling those duties. (For example, make sure board members realize that although most states limit the liability of individual board members, those waivers are based on the premise that board members have done everything they can to be prudent in their decision making.)

- **Encourage "name dropping."** Inform your board members that their friends and associates can be important to your organization. Ask members for names of potential big donors they know personally or know about.

- **Provide fund-raising training.** Just because your board is expected to help fund-raise does not mean its members know how to do it. Consider hiring a fund-raising consultant to help train and educate the board about soliciting donations. Asking for money is inherently difficult for most people. Be sure to provide customized training and role-playing exercises before launching any new fund-raising campaign.

- **Be clear about contributions.** You may feel awkward about asking your board members for money, but you cannot expect them to make a financial contribution to your

organization if they do not know what is expected
(see Putting Their Money Where Their Mouths Are,
below, for details on board member contributions.)

■ Help them put their best foot forward. Not all board
members have the same skills and interests. There
is plenty to do for your fund-raising campaign,
so match the jobs to the members.

■ Hold a board retreat. If you have not held a board
retreat in the last year, consider planning one to
invigorate your board, review progress, and analyze
current situations (see appendix B).

■ To further empower and educate your board, make
sure you have them read this manual, particularly
the information on board participation.

Explaining What to Do

Provide your board members with a detailed list of their fund-raising responsibilities (below).
Be sure to set clear expectations about fund-raising when recruiting new board members.

Board responsibilities in fund-raising:

■ Approve the organization's mission, position, and case
statements. To be effective and motivated advocates and
fund-raisers, board members must be intimately involved
in preparing these fundamental and public statements.

■ Participate in creating and approving a development
(fund-raising) plan, process, and budget. This also
includes assigning a leader and development committee
for the fund-raising program as well as board member
participation on fund-raising committees.

■ Achieve 100 percent giving from all board members (see
Putting Their Money Where Their Mouths Are, below).

■ Identify and cultivate new prospects. Each board
member should identify individual, corporate,
and foundation donors he can approach.

■ Be an advocate for the organization. Expect each board
member to use his knowledge, understanding,
and personal networks to spread the word about your
organization in an effort to garner additional support.

■ Accompany staff on key visits to supporters. Attendance
at donor cultivation visits and events is critical to building
a strong donor base. Board members should make
introductions for staff to follow up.

- Send a personal "thank you." When one of your board members takes time to personally thank a donor, it sends a powerful message about how much the organization values that donor's support.

Remember, fund-raising is friend-raising, and the board is your link to the community at large. The board that works in a positive way with the executive director, staff, and development volunteers can create a dynamic fund-raising team to fulfill the mission of the organization and provide funding for current and future programs.

Learning Your Gs, Ds, and Ws

Three sets of triplicate letters can help your board members recall particular expectations tied to their service:

- "The 3 Ds" refers to the legal obligations of board members: duty of care, duty of obedience, and duty of loyalty. These duties indicate that a good board member makes prudent decisions, respects laws and the organization's legal documents, and does not put personal interests above the interests of the organization.

- "The 3 Gs" are "give, get, or go." Many boards expect their members to bring in money by making a personal contribution or participating in fund-raising or both. If this does not happen, a board member may be asked to leave to give the seat to someone else.

- "The 3 Ws" are wealth, work, and wisdom. Besides participating in securing finances (wealth), board members are expected to participate in activities (work). The final important contribution is each board member's knowledge and expertise (wisdom).

Putting Their Money Where Their Mouths Are

Table 5.1
Expectations of Board Member Giving

Organizations requiring board members to make a personal contribution	48%
Organizations with 100 percent participation by their board	36%

Source: www.boardsource.org
(citing a National Council of Nonprofit Boards/Stanford University survey).

When you raise funds, you start with those closest to your organization and work outward, starting with your board. It is critical that every member of your board of directors makes an annual personal contribution to the organization. If any of them doesn't, potential donors will wonder why they should give you their money if those closest to your organization cannot demonstrate confidence through financial support. Major financial support from your board establishes your organization's credibility with other donors (Table 5.1).

How much should a board member give? Your goal is to achieve 100 percent giving by the board and for each board member to make a "generous" gift. Serving on your board is not a job just for the wealthy. The size of the financial contribution should depend on each member's personal financial situation.

If your board members are not giving, your board's leadership (especially the chair or president) should find out why. Do they understand their responsibilities? Are they under the misconception that their time and effort should count as their donation? Find out whether there is something tangible or emotional that is preventing board members from contributing. Then work with your board to resolve any misconceptions or underlying problem.

Opening the Lines of Communication

To become effective fund-raisers, your board needs the commitment and support of your animal care organization's staff and volunteers. Make sure your staff and volunteers understand that, although they may not be calling on donors themselves, fund-raising and friend-raising is the job of every single person in the organization.

Communicate to the entire staff the role and practices of the development department. Too often, staffs not directly involved in fund-raising have an overly simplistic view of how to raise money by relying on the sale of hats, T-shirts, or stickers. At the same time, make sure front-line staff members understand the role they play in generating goodwill and developing donor relations.

Different people from different parts of your organization will be working on your fund-raising program. If these individuals do not keep each other abreast of what they are doing, important details will fall through the cracks. Keeping lines of communication open helps your board, staff, and volunteers understand just who can solicit gifts in your organization's name and how to go about it. Make sure everyone involved in a fund-raising activity, no matter how small the venture, knows to get approval from the development department. For example, your kennel staff should not approach small businesses or individuals for help with projects unless approval was sought and received.

Staff responsibilities in fund-raising:

- Support the board in its fund-raising duties.

- Assist with creating fund-raising program materials.

- Research and track new, existing, and former donors.

- Help coordinate direct mail and letters (or phone calls or e-mails) of appreciation.

- Write grant proposals.

- Participate in fund-raising events and direct solicitations, when appropriate.

- Accompany board members on important donor cultivation visits and events.

- Be polite to all public visitors and callers—they may already be (or could be) donors.

Finding Out Who Is in Charge

Although everyone in your organization must participate in fund-raising, one person should oversee your fund-raising program. In smaller organizations, this person may be a qualified volunteer or the executive director. Many animal care organizations, however, delegate this responsibility to a full-time fund-raising professional.

Hiring a director of development does not come cheaply. These much sought-after fund-raising professionals can demand a relatively high salary. Sometimes that salary exceeds even that of his boss—the executive director—just as a professional athlete earns more than his coach. This can create some management challenges. But decision makers should remember that a good fund-raising professional can make up for higher costs by helping your organization build and carry out a successful fund-raising campaign. If your organization cannot afford a full-time director of development, consider hiring someone part time.

Your director of development should not be charged exclusively with directly soliciting funds from prospects. He at times may solicit support from event sponsors, animal-related businesses, grant-making organizations, and individuals asking how to contribute. The responsibility of soliciting major gifts rests with your board members, close supporters, and particular volunteers with established connections. The director of development creates and manages the fund-raising program through overseeing prospect files, organizing site visits, and coordinating other behind-the-scenes activities.

Here is what to look for in a director of development:

- someone with experience in nonprofit fund-raising, ideally in the animal care field

- someone with proven management and organization skills

- someone with excellent written and verbal communication skills

- someone with an engaging personality and "people skills"

- someone who can be satisfied working behind the scenes

- someone who can motivate and inspire people to raise funds

A sample job description for a director of development can be found in appendix D.6.

Involving Your Volunteers

Raising resources is not just bringing in money; it is also recruiting helping hands. When you consider all that a volunteer force brings to your organization—from hands-on program support to community animal advocacy—a trained, committed team of volunteers can be worth its weight in gold. *Volunteer Management for Animal Care Organizations* by Betsy McFarland (Humane Society Press, 2005) can offer help in recruiting, training, and retaining volunteers.

Your organization can involve a reliable, educated pool of volunteers in its fund-raising program. Here are just a few of the many ways qualified volunteers can help:

- helping out at a special event (such as by selling T-shirts or handing out education materials)

- participating in donor visits or, for specially connected and trained volunteers, hosting a donor event

- serving on a development committee

- delivering thank-yous to donors (through letters, telephone calls, or e-mail)

The director of development and the manager of volunteers must work together to plan strategies to encourage volunteers to donate their financial resources as well as their time. Separation of the development and volunteer aspects of the organization may result in missed funding opportunities from individuals who also happen to be volunteers.

Although volunteers can be a great help to your fund-raising program, they can also be a great hindrance if they are not trained, educated, and monitored. It is your responsibility to make sure your volunteers understand your organization's role and mission, know basic fund-raising procedures and etiquette, and follow protocol (such as getting approval for fund-raising activities).

Ten Basic Responsibilities of Nonprofit Boards
(from BoardSource)

1. Determine the organization's mission and purpose. It is the board's responsibility to create and review a statement of mission and purpose that articulates the organization's goals, means, and primary constituents served.

2. Select the chief executive (e.g., executive director). Boards must reach consensus on the chief executive's responsibilities and undertake a careful search to find the most qualified individual for the position.

3. Provide proper financial oversight. The board must assist in developing the annual budget and ensuring that proper financial controls are in place.

4. Ensure adequate resources. One of the board's foremost responsibilities is to provide adequate resources for the organization to fulfill its mission.

5. Ensure legal and ethical integrity and maintain accountability. The board is ultimately responsible for ensuring adherence to legal standards and ethical norms.

6. Ensure effective organizational planning. Boards must actively participate in an overall planning process and assist in implementing and monitoring the plan's goals.

7. Recruit and orient new board members and assess board performance. All boards have a responsibility to articulate prerequisites for candidates, orient new members, and periodically and comprehensively evaluate their own performance.

8. Enhance the organization's public standing. The board should clearly articulate the organization's mission, accomplishments, and goals to the public and garner support from the community.

9. Determine, monitor, and strengthen the organization's programs and services. The board's responsibility is to determine which programs are consistent with the organization's mission and to monitor their effectiveness.

10. Support the chief executive and assess his or her performance. The board should ensure that the chief executive has the moral and professional support he or she needs to further the goals of the organization.

Individual Board Member Responsibilities
(from BoardSource)

- Attend all board and committee meetings and functions, such as special events.

- Be informed and support the organization's mission, services, policies, and programs.

- Review agenda and supporting materials prior to board and committee meetings.

- Serve on committees or task forces and offer to take on special assignments.

- Make a personal financial contribution to the organization.

- Inform others about the organization.

- Suggest possible nominees to the board who can make significant contributions to the work of the board and the organization.

- Keep up-to-date on developments in the organization's field.

- Follow conflict-of-interest and confidentiality policies.

- Refrain from making special requests of the staff.

- Assist the board in carrying out its fiduciary responsibilities, such as reviewing the organization's annual financial statements.

Personal Characteristics to Consider

(from BoardSource)

- Ability to: listen, analyze, think clearly and creatively, work well with people individually and in a group

- Willing to: prepare for and attend board and committee meetings, ask questions, take responsibility and follow through on a given assignment, contribute personal and financial resources in a generous way according to circumstances, open doors in the community, evaluate oneself

- Develop certain skills if you do not already possess them, such as to: cultivate and solicit funds, cultivate and recruit board members and other volunteers, read and understand financial statements, learn more about the substantive program area of the organization

- Possess: honesty, sensitivity to and tolerance of differing views, a friendly, responsive, and patient approach, community-building skills, a developed sense of values, concern for your nonprofit's development, a sense of humor

Desired Skills, Experiences, and Qualities of Board Members

Skills and experience:

- financial management

- organizational management

- business administration

- accounting

- banking and trusts

- estate planning

- investments

- fund-raising

- law

- marketing

- human resources

- architectural planning

- engineering

- strategic or long-range planning

- business ownership

- public relations

- advertising

- philanthropy

- real estate

Look in your community for those who have a good reputation, who are active with other organizations, and who possess the qualities, attributes, and skills you seek. It is usually the busiest person who will get the job done, so start at the top. Along with a balanced set of skills, also strive for a balance in age, sex, race/ethnic background, and geographic location.

When identifying and recruiting board members, consider well-known people who will lend their names; up-and-coming community leaders who are not already overcommitted; well-positioned community leaders; upper- and mid-level managers of corporations; or active spouses and other family members of well-established leaders in the community willing to contribute "wealth, wisdom, and work" and able to "give it, get it, or go."

Getting on the Major-Gift List: How to Develop the Relations to Draw Large Donations

If your animal care organization struggles to keep track of its coin banks displayed at local retail shops, then chances are it is not ready to dive into a major-gift campaign. Make sure you can answer yes to the questions in the checklist below before launching a formal major-gifts program. (A "major gift," as defined by the Association of Fundraising Professionals, is "a significant donation to a not-for-profit organization, the amount required to qualify as a major gift determined by the organization.")

- Can you articulate your animal care organization's vision, and mission clearly to donors and the general public?

- Is your work guided by a strategic plan and development plan?

- Do you keep records of all donations by the method they came in?

- Do you send thank-you notes to donors within forty-eight hours of receiving their gifts?

- Do board members make a personal thank-you call to donors who make major gifts?

- Do you send donors an annual summary of their contributions for tax purposes?

- Do your newsletters (mailed and online) include a reminder to donors to remember your organization in their wills?

- Do you mail out one or more donor solicitations each year?

Your $10 and $20 donors need to be confident that your development program is competently managed before they can trust your organization to put larger amounts of money to good use. If you answered yes to the questions above and have fund-raising fundamentals in place, then it is time to seek a little extra from those able to give a little more.

Minor Givers *Are* Your Major Givers

As you begin to focus on major gifts, do not lose sight of the fact that every donor, no matter how large or small his gift, is of major importance to the continuation of your animal care organization. Few organizations could survive without the financial and moral support of their $10 and $20 contributors.

You may not realize it, but you are developing a major-gifts program even if you are not actively asking for gifts much bigger than those $20 checks. That's because the donors you seek now can grow into your major donors later. In fact, most major donors don't start out as major donors. It is more likely that they will start as new donors, become repeat donors, and then gradually increase the level of their giving as their interest and confidence in your organization increases.

To grow that interest and confidence, you need to show your donors that you are interested and confident in them. Get to know your donors. Who are they? Why do they give to your organization? What motivates them? What are their charity goals? What can you offer them to help meet these goals? To convince people to contribute to your organization, you need to learn more about what makes them tick. According to the Independent Sector, 57 percent of households were asked to contribute in 2000 (Table 6.1). Of these households, 61 percent actually contributed when asked, compared to 39 percent of households that were not asked.

Table 6.1

Giving in the United States, 2000

Giving in the United States, 2000	
Percentage of households contributing to charity	89
Average annual household contribution*	$1,620
Percentage of household income given*	3.1
Average contribution among volunteering households*	$2,295
Percentage of households asked to give	57
Percentage of households that gave when asked	61

Based on contributing households only.
Source: Independent Sector 2001.

Prospecting for Golden Donors

Your first chance to learn more about your donors is when you are looking for them. This is called prospecting—the systematic acquisition and recording of data about donors and prospects. It is key to your major-gifts program and your entire development program. This information forms the basis for establishing, maintaining, and expanding the long-term gift relationship with the ultimate goal of converting donors into major-gift givers.

During your prospect research, you will identify, interview, and involve potential donors to your animal care organization. Begin by checking in-house files for attendees at events, program participants, and current and past donors who can be upgraded. Valuable tidbits can be gleaned from many sources: personal conversations and interviews, donor surveys, and conversations at special events and meetings.

Design a prospect profile worksheet form that provides contact information; biographical data; business history; giving history with your organization; cultivation and solicitation contact records; publicly available contributions to other organizations; a list of information sources already checked;

and individual or foundation interests. Start by developing prospect profiles on board members and other major donors to help identify connections to other prospects.

Your goal is to collect the kind of information that helps you establish a connection with each prospect. For example, people are most willing to provide financial support when they feel involved. So identify the type of cultivation and volunteer opportunities most likely to engage the prospect.

Avoiding Information Overload

To put what you learn to good use, you need to put it where you can find it and categorize it so you can use it.

Let's say that in 2002 Mrs. Jocelyn English gave your animal care organization $1,500 in memory of her dearly missed dachshund, Dolly. She has not given money to your organization since that one-time contribution. Where is this information? How do you classify it? What do you do with it?

Your records must be organized to allow you to identify gifts and their amounts. Review cumulative and single largest gifts to arrange your donor list from highest to lowest gifts. You may have the option of outsourcing analysis of your donor file to your direct-mail vendor. This analysis can demonstrate the lifetime value of your donors and help you glean other useful details.

As you collect and categorize donor information, do not fall into the common trap of narrowing your focus to prominent community leaders and philanthropists as major-gift prospects. Just because certain people have the means does not necessarily make your organization a good fit for them. Look for people who have an interest in your organization and its mission.

Consider upgrading your organization's fund-raising software to improve your ability to analyze giving history and patterns and to generate information to strengthen development activities. Fund-raising software acts as the "memory" of the organization's fund-raising activities and its importance cannot be overlooked. For guidelines on what to look for and where to get it, see appendix D.7.

Remember, too, that records about individuals and organizations must be kept confidential and used only by appropriate staff members and trained volunteers. It is the ethical responsibility of the organization to use appropriate research methods, sources, and types of information. (For more information on legal and ethical requirements, see chapter 4.)

Getting Lost in Translation

If you are having trouble screening and ranking your prospects and top donors, seek the help of advisors from different segments of your community. Ask them to suggest prospects you may have overlooked and listen to their advice on the best way to solicit. These advisors should not be hard to find. They can include staff who have researched and worked with donors and prospects; board members; committee members; other close friends of your organization; and friends who can share information about specific segments of the community.

It is easy to become overwhelmed with this research, so break it into manageable chunks of time and information. Try to designate time each week for this project and set weekly goals. Approach research as a means of getting to know your donors and prospects in ways that help build meaningful, mutually beneficial relationships and provide avenues to contribute to your mission.

Playing Matchmaker for Major Donors

After identifying and researching your major donors and prospects, match them to fundable projects detailed in your strategic plan. Start this matching process with those already involved in your organization, such as board members, program participants, and past and current donors. Next, reach out to other individuals and institutions, particularly those whose giving priorities match your programmatic focus, including those served indirectly by your work. For example, if your organization needs a van to transport animals to adoption outreach locations, your research can help identify potential major donors with specified interest in adoption programs.

A good salesperson strives to find the right product to meet his customer's needs. He needs to understand how both the product and the customers work. You, too, must be able to sell your organization and the selected program, so make sure you can clearly explain how the work of your organization improves the quality of life in your community. Selling does not involve just talking and promoting; it involves a lot of listening to learn what the customer wants. The same holds true in fund-raising: listening is one of the most important tools in cultivating major gifts.

Take advantage of this tool by asking one of your donors to host a small-group gathering that focuses on her favored project. This person should invite other donors, friends, and prospects to a short presentation about that project, followed by a question-and-answer session. This small-group format allows you to learn more about the guests as you listen to their questions and concerns.

Establishing a Connection

Follow up by scheduling personal visits to learn even more about the interests of your individual prospects and donors. People contribute primarily to satisfy emotional needs. Personal visits can help build this emotional connection and are among the most successful ways to build depth in your development program.

Before you can ask for a major gift, you must discover what is important emotionally to the donor. You must ask a full range of questions in the discovery process, such as: What makes this important to you? Can you give me an example? What have you done in the past? How long have you been thinking about this?

Do not just nod your head politely—listen carefully and record the answers.

Although it is essential to listen to the potential donor and respond to her interests, never let the donor's offer of big money dictate the program it funds. The major donor may hold the purse strings, but you hold the knowledge, experience, and responsibility for the animals. It is up to you to educate the donor. For example, a major-gift donor, witnessing how his elderly mother perks up when he brings his dog, approaches XYZ Humane Society with a proposal to sponsor an expansive nursing-home visitation program. XYZ Humane Society does not operate this type of program and does not have the staff, time, or operational policies in place to develop and run such a program safely, humanely, and effectively. The XYZ Humane Society explains the situation to the prospective donor and tells him about a different type of outreach program that may interest him. The donor then agrees to contribute, in his mother's name, to the organization's existing humane education program in a poor neighborhood.

Broaching the Money Topic

Once you have made this connection, the next step is to find out what the donor is willing to contribute. Here you are looking for the big picture, not the details. Of course, discussing money issues is not always easy; here are some discussion points to get you started:

- "Let me ask you a question about the size of gift you are considering. What range are we talking about, assuming we can satisfy what we discussed earlier?"

- "Can we talk for a few minutes about the dollar range you are considering for your gift?"

- "Do you have any thoughts about how you'd like to make the gift?"

- "Can we talk about some numbers?"

- "There are a lot of details to cover yet. Are you comfortable talking about a gift range now and filling in details later?"

You will need to learn all you can about the prospective donor's decision-making process. For example, even if a love for animals makes the prospective donor eager to make a large gift to your organization, you may need to involve the spouse, who handles all financial decisions. To find out who and what is involved in the prospective donor's decision, consider these discussion questions:

- "Let's talk about the steps you'll take to make this decision."

- "Are you going to talk to several advisors or family members and then make a final decision?"

- "Can we talk about all the people who will be involved so we can be sure to understand any issues they may have?"

Questions can sometimes sound harsh and intrusive, so try these nurturing phrases to introduce them:

- "Help me understand better…"

- "I'd like to hear more about that. Can I ask…?"

- "Can you help me clarify something…?"

After you summarize the topics you discussed, briefly review all of the points. Then ask the donor what else she wants to talk about. If this is the last visit before you prepare a presentation to ask for the major gift, you can establish expectations by ending with a statement such as, "I think we have a good understanding of what you'd like to accomplish with a gift to us. What I'd like to do is to review the issues and present a proposal that details how we can provide an opportunity you can get excited about."

Normally, it will take approximately five personal contacts with a donor or prospect before you make the "ask" for a major gift. After completing these visits and making the right program or project match, prepare a proposal identifying the project and the amount of money requested. Build these donor-centered presentations around the donors' or prospects' major interests—you must draw the connection between their passion and your organization.

A donor will be more receptive to your proposal if you describe the gift-giving opportunity as a way for the donor to "realize a dream." Check each prospect's financial data and giving patterns before deciding the highest realistic amount of the "ask" and review the prospect's affiliations before selecting the appropriate person to do the "ask."

Sample Objections and Responses

1. **Objection:** "I'm not as wealthy as those folks who make those huge gifts you always read about."

   Response: This person may be concerned about recognition or making an impact. He may feel like a "small fish in a big pond." Try one of these responses: "Every gift is important to us regardless of magnitude. Only with the help of many caring friends joining together can we achieve our important goal" or "It is obvious that what you are considering is most generous and will have a profound impact. It's not really a matter of the dollar level but rather the use of funds to make an impact on lives that counts. In that respect, your gift is of particular significance."

2. **Objection:** "I'll do something, but I really can't do what you're asking."

   Response: Will your response differ depending on your degree of confidence in the prospect's ability to give as requested? If the prospect is capable of doing what you are asking, consider whether your cultivation attempts were adequate—perhaps your organization is not high enough on the candidate's priority list. It is possible to ask for too much, too soon, and the candidate's objection may reflect that. Does the prospect appear dispassionate or unenthusiastic? If so, try "selling the dream" but avoid price haggling at this point. You can always discuss figures another day.

Consider telling the prospect, "We deeply appreciate your support and consideration of this opportunity. Whatever you decide to give will be greatly appreciated, but we would feel remiss if we failed to present how this exciting opportunity can make a huge difference in the life of others. It is a lot to consider, and I'll plan to give you a call next Thursday to answer any questions you have and to discuss the next step in the process. I'll look forward to hearing from you."

Thanking Them Again and Again

Receiving the gift is not the end of the process. You must recognize the significance of a gift by responding immediately to the donor in ways that match the significance of the gift. Send one or more thank-you letters from the peer solicitor, the development staff, the executive director or CEO, and the board president.

Depending on the significance of the gift, consider following the thank-you letter with a phone call or personal visit. A call from a volunteer board member will have a greater impact on a donor than a call from paid staff.

Your development team is responsible for retaining your animal care organization's donors through responsible stewardship; this involves recording and tracking contributions to ensure they are used exactly as the donor intended. Make sure your development team has a system in place to track, report, and personalize gift acknowledgments so your organization can retain donors and ensure future support.

Reporting to donors how gifts were used provides a wonderful opportunity to reinforce your appreciation for a gift, fulfill your stewardship responsibilities, and position your organization for the next gift.

Chapter 7

Delivering the Mail: How to Create a Successful Direct-Mail Campaign

If you have a mailbox, you know all about the fund-raising method known as "direct mail." Like most Americans, each day you likely receive what are unfavorably labeled "give me" letters, most of which you probably toss without opening. But some catch your eye, and these you open. Maybe you recognize the name of the charity. Or perhaps there is a catchy phrase outside or bulky item inside that piques your curiosity. Of those few letters that you open and read, fewer still tempt you to pull out your wallet.

What makes you throw out certain fund-raising appeals? What causes you to open others? Most important, what entices you to write a check for a select few? Now that you are switching roles from recipient to sender, your goal is to do all you can to make sure that the fund-raising appeals that land in mailboxes like yours get transferred to "bills to be paid" pile instead of the recycle bin.

In these days of information overload, it is increasingly harder for direct-mail pieces to get noticed. Unlike bills, which demand attention, donation requests cannot compel anyone to respond. As a result, nonprofits like yours struggle to find ways to get people to open the envelopes and their checkbooks. Some groups add catchy "teasers" (provocative questions or catchphrases) to the envelopes and fill the inside with address labels, notepads, decals, pens, and even coins to win a second look.

Do Not Give Up!

If it is so hard to get people even to open your organization's mail, why go to all the expense and effort? Why not focus on other fund-raising approaches like special events, planned giving, major gifts, foundation grants, and even capital campaigns? You can and should include these fund-raisers in your development plan, but know that they all have one thing in common: they depend on a solid, systematic, successful direct-mail campaign. Simply put, effective direct mail is a foundation of your fund-raising efforts.

Developing your organization's direct-mail campaign can be challenging, but getting favorable responses from recipients is not as hopeless as your own mailbox may suggest. In fact, direct mail can help your animal care organization reach potential new donors, renew and upgrade existing donors, and focus on specific target groups. Although some may argue that direct mail is overused and lacks originality, this system remains the best way to reach a large number of people, for both fund-raising and education. Tables 7.1 and 7.2 present survey data on what factors prompt donors to open mail as well as data on how many actually respond to direct mail received.

The $10 checks you initially receive may seem insignificant, but you will find that many of those small-sum contributors later become board members and major-gift donors. Direct mail is where it all begins.

This holds true for small, underfunded nonprofits, too. Many animal care organizations feel that their small size and relatively modest budgets can be a disadvantage in direct-mail fund-raising and, in some areas, they clearly can. But being small can also have strong advantages in fund-raising, including the direct-mail component:

- A relatively small animal care organization can be in touch more closely with its donors.

- Many donors prefer supporting a smaller nonprofit, where they feel their gifts can have a greater impact than they would have at a larger nonprofit.

- Many donors prefer to donate to their community's nonprofits that provide local and direct service, such as animal care and rescue.

Table 7.1

Direct Mail Has Impact

A Vertis survey of 2,000 adults, conducted in 2003, found:	
Donors most likely to donate to an organization from which they received direct mail	59%
Donors who said that they read fund-raising and nonprofit direct mail	53%
What is the most important factor in deciding what mail to open?	
Personalized mail	62%
Timing of the mail	59%
A free gift	32%
A special offer	31%
Dated material	30%

Source: Vertis 2004.

Table 7.2

Adults Who Said They Had Responded to Direct Mail in the Last 30 Days, by Percentage

2003	46%
2001	34%

Source: Vertis 2003.

Ask and You Shall Receive

As you create your direct-mail system, keep these basic fund-raising principles prominent in the development process:

- People give because they are asked.

- People give to people.

- People respond to a winning cause.

- Donors respond to specific requests for support.

- Most donors want, and all donors deserve, recognition for their gifts.

- Enthusiasm is contagious.

That first principle—"people give because they are asked"—may seem obvious, but it is often overlooked by animal care organizations. These nonprofits often fail to ask often enough or make it easy for people to contribute. Before you dismiss this as a problem plaguing "other organizations, not mine," take a closer look around. For example, are contribution return envelopes available:

- in every direct mail piece?

- in each newsletter?

- in every non-fund-raising mailing?

- at each of your events?

- at the entrance to your shelter?

- at any public venue that attracts potential contributors?

It is simple but true: the more contribution envelopes you make available, the more needed funds you will secure.

Finding Your Footing First

You may be anxious to collect money from the thousands of citizens in your community by blanketing the whole town with direct-mail pieces. But you will end up losing more money and credibility than you gain if you do not temper that impatience with prudence. For one thing, sending out the most pieces to the most people is not going to get you the most money. Your mailing list cannot be the local telephone directory; to gain donations and support, you need to develop target mailings to a strategically developed list of potential supporters. Those mailings must reflect your organization's message, mission, professionalism, and reputation. Before you draft any of your own direct-mail pieces, collect some samples—especially from successful animal care organizations—and keep a file of the good examples, such as those in the appendices to this manual.

An effective direct-mail fund-raising campaign requires that you spend money to make money. So make sure your development plan budget contains the necessary start-up funds for a direct-mail program. Include costs associated with staff time, printing, postage, assembly (mail house), consultants, and list rental.

Many small nonprofits begin a direct-mail program only to give it up after losing money in their first few mailings. Before you give in to this temptation, keep this in mind: $100 million nonprofit organizations have begun with modest direct-mail programs. Acquiring new donors may require an initial investment that will exceed donation revenue. Do not think of this as "losing money" but as investing in your future. In fact, a lower response rate to your prospect mailing list may be successful if the average gift is higher than expected.

Grizzard Communications, a direct-mail company that works with many nonprofits, says a response rate of 1.5 percent to 2.5 percent can be anticipated when mailing to prospects. The more targeted the list, the higher response rate one can typically expect. However, like all animal care work, a successful, money-generating, direct-mail program takes patience, dedication, and a long-term commitment.

Make sure you have the people and skills necessary to develop a direct-mail program that will generate revenue, not rejection. If financially feasible, consider outsourcing direct-mail services to an experienced, qualified vendor to enable your internal development team to focus on other critical fund-raising responsibilities. Even if your team of staff, volunteers, and board members contains writers, graphic artists, list managers, and development software users, you should still consider hiring a professional consultant experienced in developing and carrying out direct-mail marketing strategies. For advice on hiring a consultant, see chapter 11.

Getting Ready for the Mail Carrier

After you have done your initial research, set your budget, and found your people, you are ready to take the eight basic steps to setting up and launching your animal care organization's direct-mail program. They are:

1. Set up the basics.

2. Identify your mailing list.

3. Develop a solicitation strategy.

4. Decide on your message.

5. Put it all together and send it out.

6. Thank donors and maintain contact.

7. Track and evaluate your mailing.

8. Solicit again.

1. Set Up the Basics

Not quite sure where your local post office is? Then you have work to do. For your direct-mail program to succeed, it is critical that you establish a good relationship with your local post office. (Your direct-mail professional or firm, if you are hiring one, already works closely with the postal service.)

If your organization does not already have a "bulk mail account," the local post office will help you set one up. Bulk mail costs considerably less than first-class mail and gets to local addresses fairly quickly. Your post office can also tell you how to set up a "business reply envelope" account. Business reply envelopes (BREs) are postage-paid return envelopes that enable contributors to mail you their donations without having to put a stamp on the envelope. Although this makes it easier for donors to contribute, many animal care organizations include a line on the envelope that says, "Your first-class stamp helps us help more animals," whereby the donor pays postage so the nonprofit organization does not have to.

Postal employees can also advise you on the direct-mail piece itself. Any non-standard pieces—odd shapes and sizes, colors, and different weights—can change your postage rates. Before mass-producing and mass-mailing anything, take a mock-up to the post office. You do not want to spend time and money creating a masterpiece only to find out that it will be absurdly expensive to mail or, worse yet, cannot be mailed at all. (And no, you cannot count on your designer or graphic artist to know the ins and outs of the latest postal regulations.)

Postal regulations aren't the only requirements you will need to explore before embarking on your direct-mail program. If your organization has not yet registered in your state (and, if applicable, other states), contact the appropriate state agency (usually the Secretary of State or the office of the Attorney General). Those new to direct mailing often get into trouble because they did not check with the post office or register with the appropriate state agency. A little forethought and preparation can save you a bundle in unexpected and unnecessary fees.

The next door you will need to knock on is a printer's. The printing business is extremely competitive, and that works in your favor. So do not hand this large printing job to the XYZ Printing Company just because you have used that company for years. Instead, solicit bids from several firms to find the best deal (and to find a backup printer if you run into problems later). Ask, too, about price breaks for volume orders. For example, you may be able to save a lot of money by placing one order for a year's supply of reply envelopes instead of placing separate orders for each mailing.

Depending on the size and complexity of your mailing, you may need to find a "mail house"—a company that assembles your direct-mail piece. It is tempting to try to save money by putting everything together yourself with assistance from dedicated volunteers. But a team of your best volunteers still lacks the speed and accuracy of a competent, professional mail house. For large mailings, volunteer time taken up by stuffing envelopes means less time spent on other worthy programs. On the other hand, small groups using volunteers for a mailer of five hundred to a thousand pieces can be cost-effective for the organization and meaningful for those who participate.

As you set up this compilation and distribution system, do not neglect to set up a firm production timeline and mailing schedule. You do not want to spend lots of resources creating a spectacular winter-holiday package only to have it arrive to prospects in January. And you do not want your attractive announcement of a special event to arrive after the event. Make sure that designers, printers, and mail-service providers work cooperatively and stick to an agreed-upon timeline.

Many direct-mail service providers want your business, but their professionalism and expertise can vary considerably. As you look for help externally, use caution, check references, and avoid long-term contracts.

2. Identify Your Mailing List

After your basic setup is complete, you are ready to decide who will receive your mailings. Selecting the right list is one of the most critical components of a successful direct-mail program. Divide your selection into two basic groups:

- Your house file. These are your current donors, so they are easy to identify.

- Your prospect or acquisition list. These are your potential donors (such as adopters, people who surrender animals, volunteers, etc.). Ask your animal care organization's board members, volunteers, and other supporters to suggest people who may be interested in supporting or learning more about your organization. Strive to include anyone who has had positive contact with your organization.

Also consider working with a direct-mail list broker who will rent your organization a list of names of people likely to support your organization. Although list prices vary, you can generally expect to pay in the range of five to ten cents per name, depending on the number of names rented and the type and quality of the list. Generally, most list brokers will not deal with quantities of fewer than five thousand names, and many deal only with much larger quantities. (To find a broker, ask other local nonprofits, a direct-mail consultant, or mail house.)

Response lists consisting of supporters of other (local and national) humane organizations; other nonprofits with similar but unrelated missions; magazine subscribers; and consumer lists (catalog and Internet) work far better than do compiled lists based solely on demographic information (such as household zip codes). According to Mike Monk, vice president of Grizzard Communications, your organization should strive to have 8 percent to 10 percent of potential households in your market on your donor file.

3. Develop a Solicitation Strategy

Generally, the more you mail, the better you do. But the more you mail, the more money it costs. So with limited resources you will have to be selective. Focus first on your best donors and prospects and send them mailings frequently. You need to strike a balance between enough and too much. Many organizations make the mistake of sending mailings too infrequently, failing to heed the advice, "If you don't ask people won't give." On the other hand, organizations that send mailings out every other week risk draining their funds and irritating potential donors.

This solicitation strategy must correlate with your budget and include realistic income expectations. Everyone involved in carrying out or signing off on fund-raising activities must understand that direct mail can be expensive, especially if your organization buys lists or goes prospecting. Initially return rates may vary and often are very low. You may not net any return at all. For example, if the response rate is 1 percent to 3 percent of the total number of pieces mailed out, or the response does not show a net, explain to your board that a 2 percent response is considered excellent or that no net was expected. Before mailing any direct-mail piece, your development department must provide reasonable expectations on returns, which can vary depending on whether the organization is mailing to major donors, its own mailing list, a purchased list, a "cold" list, all residents, or other groupings. To determine if a particular mailing is successful, income, net, percentage returns, percentage new donors, and percentage of upgraded donors all need to be projected.

Make sure everyone understands the realities of launching an ambitious program. You do not want uninformed board members and other leaders to balk halfway through your campaign because they didn't understand that it is common to lose money in the beginning. Educate your team that a successful solicitation strategy requires a goal to secure contributors, not dollars. Everyone involved in your direct-mail program must be willing to make an investment in the future.

4. Decide on Your Message

Selecting your message should be relatively easy, because you work closely with the issues. As you develop your message, keep in mind that repetition is critical. Both for fund-raising success and effective education, a good story bears repeating in an individual direct-mail appeal and in subsequent mailings. And, of course, your direct-mail piece must explain your organization's financial needs, its objectives, and the specific benefits gained through donor dollars.

Be wary of dwelling on your fiscal problems. "We will have to close our animal shelter if you don't contribute now" may work once or twice. But after a few times, that message implies that your animal care organization is poorly managed. Your organization's needs (and the needs of the animals) are important, but sounding desperate is not a long-term strategy.

Instead, be upbeat and focus on success. People respond to a winning cause and enthusiastic approach: "It's a tough battle, but with your generous support, we are helping more animals all of the time" and "We have exceeded our goal with an all-time record of support, but much still remains to be done" tells supporters and potential donors that your organization knows how to use their donations to make a real difference.

This message can include a story about how a certain animal was helped. Follow these tips to make sure that story and accompanying photographs contribute to your direct-mail goals:

- Use the animal's name.

- Avoid graphic photos and lengthy details of the rescue and rehabilitation. Move from the story to the "ask."

- Consider "before and after" photos but avoid using too many photos of sad, skinny, abused animals (this may cause the reader to conclude that these are the only animals you adopt out).

- Focus on what you did for the animal and how the donations helped. If you show and discuss an injured animal, be sure to focus, too, on the "after."

- Avoid focusing on solo animals and animals behind bars. Instead, show animals with staff and adopters. This helps communicate the partnership your organization has with both people and animals.

- Resist the temptation to show photos of dead animals to illustrate problems. Instead of motivating people to donate, these photos often immobilize the reader.

- Review the article on photographs in the January/February 2004 issue of *Animal Sheltering* magazine, which can be found at *www.animalsheltering.org*.

To attract and keep donors' respect and your organization's integrity, your message must be accurate and fair. Do not criticize other organizations in an attempt to win supporters. Language such as, "We don't kill animals like the XYZ Humane Society does," is divisive and could damage your relationships with other organizations in the community.

5. Put It All Together and Send It Out

Establishing a good message is essential, but so is the overall appearance of the piece. While you want to make sure that yours contains proper spelling and grammar, you do not want it to look and read like a college term paper or a formal business letter. To grab and keep the reader's interest, follow these tips:

- **Keep it clean and simple.** Do not attempt to cram as much text as possible on a page—you will only intimidate your reader. Instead, make your letter reader-friendly with plenty of white space and large type. (Many direct-mail contributors are older and have trouble reading small text.)

■ **Keep the letter's tone friendly and informal.** Readers should hear the voice of a like-minded person talking about his love of animals.

■ **Structure the letter with skimmers in mind.** Use bullet points, bold type, underlines, and italics. Repeat your core message several times. (To do this, a longer letter is generally better.)

■ **Use as much personalization as possible.** "Dear Friend" letters work, but computers make personalization easy. It is also nice to specifically thank someone for his last gift.

■ **Select the right person to sign the letter.** Think "name recognition"—which person representing your organization is best known in the community? For most animal care organizations, the appropriate person to sign letters will be the organization's CEO, president, or executive director. Also consider the signer's relationship with your organization. Presidents, for example, may be involved with your organization for only a short time and may not be accessible to donors wishing to discuss the solicitation.

■ **Strive for consistency.** You are trying to establish and build relationships, so demonstrate stability by keeping certain elements like the letter signer and organization logo consistent in subsequent mailings. For those who have increased their giving, however, try personalizing your approach (see next bullet item).

■ **Adjust your approach.** Scrutinize returns to identify those with consistent increased giving levels and alter mailings accordingly. These donors should receive a personalized, closed-face package with a first-class stamp. This approach can improve response rates and average gifts dramatically. In fact, in a 2003 survey (Table 7.1), 62 percent of respondents selected "personalized mail" as the most important factor in deciding what mail to open.

■ **Do not hesitate to be a name-dropper.** If your organization is fortunate enough to count among its supporters a celebrity, community leader, veterinarian, or other prominent, highly regarded person, find a way to mention that person's support in your letter.

■ **Make sure you have it all together.** Your direct-mail appeal should include the appeal letter, an envelope to put it into (called a "carrier" envelope), any premium (such as address labels or notepads), a reply card, and a reply envelope. (Instead of enclosing both a reply card and a reply envelope, many organizations insert a long-

Fund-Raising for Animal Care Organizations

flapped envelope that combines the two pieces. Such consolidation can save the organization money and reduce the number of pieces the mail house, donor, and development office must handle (or lose).

- **Double-check that reply envelope.** Sometimes the most obvious and important things are overlooked. Your job is to make it easy for people to support your shelter. If they have to work too hard to figure out how to send you a check, they may opt for the easy way out by tossing your mailing.

- **Request donor details.** Most people will not bother to give you their e-mail addresses, phone numbers, and employer information. But if your reply slip requests this useful information, some people will provide it.

- **Consider putting in a little extra.** Many animal care organizations place "premiums"—free items—in their direct mail. Examples include pens, personalized address labels, and greeting cards. Basic premiums are inexpensive, but cost effective only in larger quantities. If your direct-mail program is in its infancy or consists of small quantities, hold off on using premiums until it becomes more established. Many organizations find that including these premiums pays off—especially early in the acquisition period. Keep in mind, however, that not all potential supporters like premiums. Some recipients get bored and overwhelmed with common freebies (like personalized address labels). Other people do not like to see organizations they support spend money on "junk" that could go to worthy programs instead.

- **Remember to ask for a gift!** Your letter may provide a wonderfully convincing testimonial about your organization's good work on behalf of both animals and people in your community. But if you do not ask directly and clearly for money and support, you will not get any. Ask for a gift early in the appeal letter and repeat the request at least once.

Sending your mailing sounds simple enough, but for some it can be the most difficult part of the entire process. Generally, people hate to ask for money, even if they care deeply about the animals. Consequently, the last thing that often happens at an animal care organization is sending out direct mail. At some point you must stop deliberating on the message and get your direct-mail piece written, designed, assembled, and sent (see appendix D.8 for sample direct mail pieces). The only sure way to guarantee that you will not receive any donations from your mailing is to not to send it out in the first place.

6. Thank Donors and Maintain Contact

You have received a gift, now what do you do? Thank the contributor! Every contributor should be thanked, regardless of the gift amount. Follow these thank-you tips to keep in your donors' good graces:

- **Consider different methods.** A thank-you letter is a classic way to thank a contributor (and it gives you a chance to ask for another gift). But it is also effective and acceptable to thank the giver with a simple e-mail or quick phone call (a great job for a volunteer).

- **Thank and thank again.** Generally, the more often (and the more personally) you thank a contributor, the better the long-term relationship.

- **Consider your future.** Do not neglect those $10 contributors. Large contributors almost always begin as modest contributors, so thanking every contributor effectively is not just the right thing to do, it is the smart thing to do.

- **Get help from above.** A simple way to start cultivating larger donations is to have your executive director or president call and thank all donors who contributed above a specific amount determined by your organization.

- **Add a personal touch.** Donors may feel unappreciated if this year's thank-you letter looks identical to the one received last year or if the text and signature appears too generic. Sometimes it is all you can do even to get generic thank-you letters out. But, whenever possible, strive to vary letter content and personalize your thank-you letters.

- **Make them famous.** Creating donor "honor rolls" or "walls of honor" are great ways to recognize your contributors formally and publicly. What's more, such acknowledgment methods can encourage more gifts. You need to respect the wishes of those donors wishing to remain anonymous, but most donors want and deserve recognition for their gifts.

7. Track and Evaluate Your Mailing

Different people respond differently to different appeals. You need to keep track of the varying responses if you want your direct-mail program to succeed. Tracking responses even on a basic level will save you money and increase your response rate. Here's what to do:

- **Avoid the black hole.** Sending multiple mailings to people who never respond gains you nothing but a dwindling bank account. Run your donor file through the National Change of Address System at least once a year; each "cleaning" service costs between $250 and $500. If certain individuals do not respond to your direct mail, remove them from your solicitation list and substitute new prospects. Also be diligent about honoring people's requests to be removed from your mail list. Monitor your system to make sure paper and postage are not being wasted on incorrect or duplicate addresses.

■ **Get out your coloring pens.** Simply marking response envelopes down the side with different color markers can give you an easy way to track results. For example, your organization can code the envelopes in its newsletter blue and in its spring direct-mail appeal red. More sophisticated methods will improve tracking, but starting with this simple method can provide basic details about what mailings work and what do not.

■ **Make use of a donor database.** A good database will make you money and save you time; a bad one—or having none at all—will cost you both. Although you can get by with such programs as Excel, Access, or Word, your organization should acquire database software specifically for fund-raising. Prices range from several thousand dollars on up. Before selecting a program, talk with other animal care organizations and nonprofits to see what they use and how they like it. For more information about fund-raising software and databases, see appendix D.7.

■ **Glean as much information as possible.** Do not just glance at those return envelopes—scrutinize them. Make sure that valuable details such as e-mail addresses and phone numbers and corrected contact information make their way into your database. The more you know about your donors, the better.

■ **Delineate the differences.** Your board will evaluate the direct-mail piece, likely critiquing content, color palette, message, and other elements. Help your board members better analyze the piece by noting the targeted recipient (segment of the community or category of donor) and explaining the purpose (soliciting help for a special project, specific animal, or annual campaign, for example). You are less likely to face criticism when all elements are understood and when the piece meets or exceeds expectations.

■ **Do not get emotionally attached.** Just because you like a particular direct-mail piece does not necessarily mean that it will work. Make sure you evaluate each mailing and heed the adage, "the numbers don't lie." If everyone at your organization loved your direct-mail piece but the returns were disappointing, then you need to change the appeal. The average direct-mail donor is a specific kind of person, and you need to direct your appeal to that individual. Continue to monitor what everyone else in the direct-mail world is doing. If it works for another animal care organization, chances are good that it will work for you.

8. Solicit Again

Ah, you are done—for the moment. Soon the direct-mail process begins all over again. Keep asking your best contributors for their support, and always ask them for increases.

How often should you ask for a gift? Obviously your time and financial resources are a limiting factor. But "not getting around to it," is not a valid reason to postpone or limit mailings. The more direct mail you send, the more needed funds you will raise. Ideally, your animal care organization should send out at least four direct-mail pieces each year (in addition to other solicitations). Certainly it is important to honor requests from donors who only want to be solicited once or twice during the year. But unless they ask for you to stop or limit mailings, assume they do not mind receiving them. If someone tells you that he is upset about the mailing, strive to engage him in a conversation to defuse his anger and enlist the person's friendship.

As you gear up for your next solicitation, consider all that goes on in and around your organization as an opportunity to educate and enlist the support of direct-mail recipients. Your development and public relations departments should work together closely to make sure current and relevant events make their way into your appeals. For example, if your organization has been involved in a major cruelty case that garnered lots of media coverage, use that story in your next direct-mail appeal to reinforce a message about the positive impact your organization has on animals and the community.

Every humane organization should do direct mail and phone-a-thons, personal, face-to-face solicitations, special events, and e-mail/web fund-raising. But exactly how, to what degree, and when you use these methods will depend on your needs, goals, resources, and budget. Certainly, no organization that expects to succeed in fund-raising can rely solely on direct mail. But direct mail remains a great way to advance a comprehensive fund-raising program. Just make sure you start with the basics. For more information on how to establish a direct-mail campaign to help your animal care organization grow and thrive, see Resources. To learn more about "direct e-mail" see chapter 12.

Chapter 8

Getting Grants: How to Appeal to Foundations

Many novice grant seekers begin their search believing that a foundation grant is free money, readily available to just about any worthy organization that asks for it. According to Foundation Giving Trends (The Foundation Center 2004), the environment and animals sub-sector received only 5.9 percent of all grant dollars given in 2002 (Figure 8.1). After receiving rejection letter after rejection letter, those grant seekers soon feel frustrated and ready to give up.

That is too bad. After all, sizeable grants can make a huge difference to those organizations willing and able to engage in the research, planning, preparation, and follow-through necessary to woo generous foundations.

Are You Ready?

Before you get out your pen and paper to draft a grant proposal, make sure your animal care organization has all it needs:

- 501(c)(3) status

- an income and expense statement (preferably an audited financial statement from the previous year)

- a board of directors willing to call and visit foundations

- an employee or a dedicated volunteer to research foundations and write proposals

- an employee or dedicated volunteer to prepare the budget

- a strategic funding plan that provides for its basic operational costs

Figure 8.1

Foundation Grant Dollars Given, by Organization Type

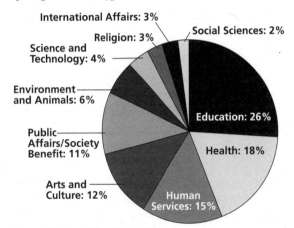

Sources: The Foundation Center 2004;
The Foundation Center's Statistical Information Service 2004.

Do not gloss over that last item. It is tempting but dangerous to view grants as life preservers for your organization. Wonderful as they are, grants are not dependable sources of income. Your organization must meet basic operating costs through contracts, membership dues, service fees, and other reasonably reliable money sources.

So before going after grant money, make sure you can afford to receive that grant money. Such money can be a great jump start for innovative special projects and enhanced services for your organizations, but until you can obtain, sustain, and protect funds for general operations and basic services, you should devote your fund-raising focus to securing financial stability.

Foundations themselves want assurance that your organization can meet basic costs on its own. If it cannot, a foundation officer may conclude that your organization will not survive. Grant givers like to give to organizations that put the money to good use and make it have lasting impact.

This makes it tough for new organizations without track records. If your organization is new, do not write off writing grant proposals. Instead, invest some time in developing relationships with foundations so they know who you are and what you do once your start-up has proven itself a capable and deserving organization.

Research: The Key to Success

It is tempting to write one grant proposal and mass-mail it to every foundation in America. But this shotgun approach will gain you only a folder full of rejection letters and little, if any, money. With the proper research, your proposals will be targeted to the interests of the specific foundation, and your chances of success will increase significantly.

Your initial research will focus on finding and honing in on foundations most likely to provide grants to your organization. As you develop your list, do not restrict yourself to those foundations that fund animal welfare. Foundations that support K–12 education, for example, may fund a humane education program. Foundations provide funding for anti-violence programs, volunteer programs, and many other projects that your organization may run. For example, the organization Senior Pets for Seniors in Brimfield, Illinois, has received grants from foundations that support projects to better the lives of senior citizens.

Sometimes the best foundations are right under your nose. Family and community foundations give entirely to organizations in the local community or region. Financially supported by individual donors in the community, these foundations are charged with providing grants to worthy local charities. These foundations strive to improve life in the local community and may assist local animal-protection organizations not just with grants but also with valuable information leading to other sources of support. (See Resources for a list of web sites identifying family foundations and community foundations.)

Although obtaining grants from foundations can be challenging, finding foundations has become easier. Here are some tips to get you started.

Roam the web. Two major web sites can help you identify foundations to approach. The Foundation Center (*www.fdncenter.org*) offers several levels of access to its database of foundations. The more foundations available to the user, the higher the cost (fees range from approximately $20 to $150). This database can be searched by state and by funding category. The listings provide a brief description of the foundation and its interests; its trustees and officers; deadlines; and suggestions on approaching the foundation (for example, whether you should send a letter of inquiry or a full proposal). The user also can access the foundation's latest Form 990, which contains such valuable information as the foundation's assets, how much money it gave away in the previous year, and which organizations it funded and at what level. Analyzing this information can tell you how much money you might reasonably request from a particular foundation. For example, a foundation's average grant may be $50,000, but its funding for animal organizations may be at the $500 level. In this case, your organization is unlikely to receive $50,000, so you need to adjust both your proposal and your expectations accordingly. The Foundation Center web site offers online tutorials in proposal writing and foundation research. The Foundation Center itself runs "bricks and mortar" libraries located in New York, Washington, D.C., Atlanta, Chicago, and San Francisco, and its publications can be found in libraries in several other cities. A visit to one of these libraries, or even a local library, may provide valuable information.

Www.guidestar.org provides a free foundation listing, which contains little information beyond the foundation's Form 990. But for an annual fee ($49/month or $499/year), GuideStar provides the user with more detailed information on the foundations.

The Foundation Center and GuideStar web sites provide the advantage of a database that you can search using keywords and other search terms. Make a list of keywords that reflect your program interests; for example, you might try "animal welfare," "education," "volunteer," or "wildlife."

It is possible, of course, simply to search the Internet for foundations using Google or a similar search engine. Many larger foundations have their own web sites containing valuable information such as a downloadable annual report and a list of recent grant recipients. Although smaller foundations may not have a web site, a search may turn up a press release from a grantee or other information that will help you understand how to interest the foundation in your work.

Get professional help. Every state has a grant makers association. These associations are umbrella organizations for foundations in that state. While they will not provide funding, they often assist organizations in writing grant proposals. They may even provide a "common grant proposal format" that is accepted by several foundations in the state.

Look closer to home. Your local library and the local chapter of the Association of Fundraising Professionals (AFP) (*www.afpnet.org*) may have a listing of local foundations. The AFP may offer programs and classes in your areas as well, such as sessions that provide an opportunity to meet local foundation officials.

Chase down recipients. Organizations that have been funded by foundations may be one of your best sources of information. Most grant recipients will not consider you a competitor because they have already been funded. You can find out which organizations a foundation has funded by reviewing the foundation's 990, examining its annual report, or conducting an Internet search.

After you track down recipients willing to share their experience, consider asking these questions:

- How do you think the foundation will respond to our program idea?

- Was there anyone at the foundation who was particularly helpful?

- How long did it take to receive funding?

- Did you receive a grant for your first application?

- If you were turned down the first time, what reason was given and how did you follow up with the foundation?

- What form did the review process take?

- Did the foundation conduct a site visit?

- Did the foundation request any additional information about your organization?

- Based on your experience, do you have any parting advice?

Be certain to thank them for their assistance!

Avoiding Information Overload

All of this research will lead to some invaluable information, including:

- list of foundations to approach

- topics and values of most interest to the foundation

- best person in your organization to make your case to the foundation

- best person at the foundation to approach

- dollar amount for your request

- application deadlines

- first step to take with that foundation: phone call, visit, letter of inquiry, or submission of full proposal

So how do you sort through the names, select those funders most likely to bestow a grant, and keep all the information organized? First, grab some folders and create a file for each funder. Then create a separate file on your computer listing each foundation, its areas of interest, and how much money you might request from the foundation (and for which program). Make another file listing the foundations by deadline so you won't miss important due dates and a chance at a generous grant.

If your board of directors is willing to approach foundations, circulate a list of each foundation's trustees and officers. Your board members may even know some of these individuals and be willing to contact them on the organization's behalf. (If your board is not willing to reach out to foundations, turn to chapter 5 for tips on getting your board involved in fund-raising.)

As you move closer to establishing relationships, recall the popular fund-raising adage, "people give to people." Even foundations are much more inclined to give when they know the players well.

Initiating the Relationship

Foundations will give your organization more consideration if they understand how your programs benefit not just local animals but everyone in the community. So one of your first missions is to show these foundations the many links between helping animals and helping people.

To make this point effectively, you need to develop a relationship with each foundation. Foundation program officers rely on their knowledge of an organization to help them determine which grants to award. That's why it is a good idea to meet with a foundation representative to summarize the proposed project and listen to feedback before submitting your full proposal. (Even a brief conversation can help your cause significantly.) This step may not guarantee approval but it makes writing the grant proposal worth the investment of time and money.

Developing a relationship can take time, so be persistent. If you are able to secure a face-to-face meeting, congratulations. During this initial meeting, explain that you want to acquaint the foundation with your organization. While you don't want to overload anyone, give the foundation representative your annual report, newsletter, and any other publications that highlight your organization's mission, programs, goals, and successes. During this short, fifteen-minute (or so) meeting, the foundation will likely determine whether its interests align with the work of your organization. It is critical, therefore, that you make the case that aiding animal-protection groups serves the entire community.

After you have laid the groundwork about your organization and its programs, ask if the foundation would be interested in receiving a proposal. If the answer is yes, do not leave without finding out what it is willing to fund—operating costs, project costs, or some other specific need—and what funding level it considers appropriate. Remember that you are building a relationship here, so always leave on a positive note.

You can still build a relationship even if the foundation is not open to face-to-face meetings or is headquartered too far away. Pick up the phone and ask to speak to a decision maker—either a program officer or the president of the foundation. Come prepared with key points you'd like to discuss as well as a memorized message in case you're connected to voice mail. Be ready to provide a thirty-second statement about your project and how it fits with the guidelines of the foundation. Explain that you think the project is a good match for the foundation and request a ten-minute conversation. If you have left messages and have not received a call back, do not feel rejected. These are busy people who may require additional calls—persistence (but not pestering) pays off.

When you do speak with the representatives, consider these discussion topics:

- their initial reaction to your program

- the importance of animal-protection issues in relation to other areas they fund

- their perception of how animal protection fits with the interests of the foundation

- ways in which the project may be framed so it is competitive with other proposals the foundation is considering

- the best time to submit your proposal (confirm printed deadlines)

- your appreciation for their time and assistance

Letter of Inquiry

If you are unable to make personal contact with the foundation, or if the foundation requests that your first contact be in the form of a letter, submit a letter of inquiry. A letter of inquiry provides a brief (two- to three-page) overview of your proposal. Sometimes foundations, even smaller foundations, will fund a project based on the letter of inquiry, but its purpose is to persuade the reader that the project is worth reviewing in more detail. A standard letter of inquiry follows this format:

In the first paragraph:

1. Identify your organization and mention any previous contact you may have had with the foundation.

2. State clearly your purpose for writing: "I am writing to inquire whether the Sandstone Community Foundation would consider a proposal for our project to conduct humane education classes in schools throughout Dallas."

3. Provide the total cost of the project and the amount requested of the foundation.

In the body of the letter:

1. State the mission of the organization and connect it to the proposed project.

2. Explain the problem or the need addressed by the proposed project.

3. Describe the project activities and explain how the project will help alleviate the need or problem.

4. Summarize the objectives that will be achieved.

In the concluding paragraph:

1. Stress how the project will be able to help alleviate the problem or need.

2. Restate the funding request. Ask if the foundation would care to see a full proposal and provide a phone number of someone who can answer any questions about the project.

3. Mention any follow-up plans you may have—such as phoning the foundation in the next two weeks.

4. Thank the foundation for considering your request.

This outline is very similar to the outline for a full grant proposal. To understand how to make the letter as effective as possible, read the section below, The Art of Persuasion.

Writing Successful Grant Proposals

It is true that the best-written proposal in the world cannot guarantee funding. But it is also true that the most deserving organization will be turned down if it cannot create a well-written, typewritten, comprehensive, persuasive proposal.

Writing a grant proposal is hard, tiring work. When you are finally finished with the first draft, it is tempting to fold it, stick it in an envelope, and head to the post office. Do this and all that hard work will likely be for nothing. Your first draft is great for brainstorming and laying out all of your ideas, but it is rarely good enough to submit to the foundation. You must take the time to revise what you have written to better construct, clarify, and condense the ideas outlined in your initial draft.

If writing is not your forte and every line of the proposal presents a struggle, consider soliciting the help of someone experienced in writing grant proposals. At the very least, have another person review your proposal before it is sent to the foundation. Do not let ego get in the way—take all criticisms seriously. After all, if your reviewers express concerns over content or style, so might the foundation's program officer.

It's easy to become so immersed in your work that you have trouble seeing it objectively. Try putting the proposal or letter aside for a day or two. Then, when you pick it up again, you will likely find fresh ways to tackle an issue or revise a problem. Creating a proposal is grueling work, but there are plenty of resources available to see you through it. The sections below walk you through the basics, and you can find additional information in Resources.

The Art of Persuasion

When you write a grant proposal, you are writing a persuasive argument. Going back to ancient times can help you write a persuasive proposal in modern times. The philosopher Aristotle noted three major elements in all arguments:

- *Ethos* is the ethical basis of your argument: why should the reader believe in you and in what you are saying?

- *Logos* is the logical reasoning underlying your argument: logic should make up the bulk of your argument.

- *Pathos* is the emotional side of your argument: pathos can be used to great effect, but only if it is used sparingly.

Ethos is emphasized in the beginning of the grant proposal where you provide background information. This basic information about your organization—the date it was founded, the number of animals served in a year, and other financial support received—allows you to argue that your organization is ethical and worthy of support. The proposal evaluator should see that your organization has established a basis for requesting funds: it is well respected in the community and has a verifiable record of achievement. Making the ethos of your argument early will prepare the reader to accept the logic of the argument that follows.

Logic will always be the deciding factor for the foundation. Be certain that your argument is developed fully, analyzed carefully, and supported by evidence. It may be tempting to skirt issues that are complex or controversial, but you want to make certain that all questions that may be raised are answered in the body of the proposal.

Once the argument has been made, a little *pathos* can be injected. Pathos is best used at the conclusion of your argument because it moves the reader to action. If you include these three elements—*ethos*, *logos*, and *pathos*—your proposal should be considered carefully by the foundation because your organization can and will do what you propose; the project will achieve an important goal for the community; and the argument makes logical sense and is fully supported by evidence. Your goal is for the reader to say, "I care about the results this project will achieve, and I will champion the proposal."

What Goes Where

If a foundation provides a suggested format for the grant proposal, use it. Program officers read through hundreds of proposals every year. You do not want readers to work hard to ferret out the information they need to judge your proposal.

The format below is one commonly accepted by foundations. It includes:

- title page

- abstract or executive summary

- organizational background

- statement of need or problem

- project description, including goals and objectives, methods and activities, management plan, staff credentials, and timeline

- sustainability plan

- evaluation

- budget

- attachments

You may not need all of these sections, or you may not go into as much detail as suggested below. What you include depends on the size and complexity of your project. Remember that bigger is not better—try to keep the proposal to no more than ten pages. It takes effort to write succinctly, but that effort should pay off in clarity.

Title Page—The title page should include the project title; the animal care organization's name and address; the contact person's name and phone number; and the proposal submission date. The title itself should be short, snappy, and memorable—make it stand out from the start.

Abstract or Executive Summary—Although the abstract appears first in the proposal, write it after completing all of the other parts of the proposal. Keep the abstract short—one page or less. This part serves two purposes: (1) to provide the hurried reader with a bite-size, digestible overview of the proposal and (2) to convince that hurried reader that the proposal is worth a more careful review. Although the material is similar, try to restate it. If the goal is to make the reader care about the project, you do not want to irritate or bore her by repeating yourself.

Organizational Background—In one page or less, you need to persuade the reader that your organization can carry out the proposed project. Here is where you will stress the rhetorical principle of *ethos*. You must demonstrate that your organization has a credible standing in the community. Depending on your organization's history, consider covering these points:

- when and by whom your organization was founded

- where your organization's financial support comes from

- what major accomplishments your organization claims

- how your work differs from the work of similar organizations

- what your organization's track record of service includes

This section provides a natural opportunity to explain why the work of your animal care organization is important to the entire community, a fact that will increase your chances of funding.

Statement of Need or Problem—The objective here is to convince the reader that the proposed project concerns a problem (pet overpopulation) or need (humane education) serious enough to warrant a response. Most persuasive arguments are built on an analysis of cause and effect. Sit down with others in your organization to brainstorm about the causes and effects of the problem. Next it is time to narrow that long list to the principal causes your proposed program is designed to help resolve. For example, if you seek funding for a feral cat trap, neuter, and return project, you might discuss the high number of cats in this country and their rate of reproduction. Because your project focuses specifically on treating the cats, you probably would not extend the argument to include irresponsible pet owners (even though they play a role in the steadily increasing feral cat population).

Here is where you will use *logos*, or logic, to make your argument persuasive. If your argument states that your project will lower pet overpopulation by trapping, neutering, and returning, persuasive evidence might include illustrative examples and national and local statistics. You might provide evidence (ideally, quoting a published source) of the estimated population of feral cats on a national level, the number of feral cats identified by your organization, and surveys or interviews with neighborhood residents and business owners.

Project Description: *Goals and Measurable Objectives*—At the beginning of the description, you need to enumerate the project's goals and measurable objectives. Here you will explain how the project will tackle the need or problem. The goal should be broad and overarching. Try writing the objectives first and then ask yourself, "Why do this?" The answer to that question should lead you to your goal.

The objectives are steps toward realizing the goal. These objectives should be specific and measurable. Remember to be realistic, but also show that the project will have a significant impact, for example:

Goal:

■ "Build a safer community by educating our children in kindness and respect for all living things."

Objectives:

■ One hundred fifty children in grades one through three at Stevensville Elementary will participate in the humane education program.

■ Seventy-five percent of the children will demonstrate gains in their knowledge of the importance of treating all living things with kindness and respect.

Typically, your project description will also contain:

■ the methods or activities used to obtain the objectives

■ a project management plan

■ the staff and their qualifications

■ the timeline

Project Description: *Methods and Activities*—Every cause has an effect; here is where you will show what effect your project will have on those causes selected in your earlier brainstorming session. Specifically, explain thoroughly how the project will create the necessary change. Prove that you have considered every major aspect of the project but do not complicate the section with too much detail. Although the complexity of the project determines the length of the section, limit it to no more than a couple of pages.

Project Description: *Management Plan*—This is the section where you will demonstrate that your organization can carry out the project. Read through your project description and make a list of the activities and the steps necessary to conduct them. Then place the steps in chronological order. You need to answer who will do what, when, where, and how. The management plan may be either a narrative or a chart; however, a chart allows you to incorporate the timeline into the management plan.

Project Description: *Staff Credentials*—For most projects, you typically will include a list of the project staff and a short description of their qualifications. For bigger projects, consider attaching resumes of key personnel.

Project Description: *Timeline*—A popular format entails listing in a table the objective, the activities needed to reach the objective, the staff person or persons responsible, and the expected date of completion. This type of format can provide the reader with a clear sense of how the project will come together. Whatever the format, keep it simple. Include all key activities, but don't burden the reader with excess detail.

Sustainability Plan—Many foundations request a "sustainability plan" that shows how the program will be funded in the future. A foundation also might ask what other sources of funding have been secured or are being sought for this project. Because foundations want their money to have maximum impact, they may choose a proposal with a good sustainability plan over those from other deserving organizations.

For many organizations, however, creating the sustainability plan can be the most difficult part of the proposal. After all, if you could afford to fund the project in the first place, you would not need to write the proposal.

Brainstorm about ways the grant can help leverage more funds for your organization. It is not enough to suggest that you will go after additional foundation funding, because securing such funding cannot be guaranteed. A sustainability plan must never begin or end with the statement that more grant proposals will be written. Instead, try to find a way to build sustainability into your project.

If your animal care organization seeks funds for its humane education program, for example, the budget might include funds for community outreach activities designed to increase support for the program. These outreach activities might encompass visits to local churches, parent-teacher associations, the Junior League, and the Chamber of Commerce to encourage these groups to "adopt a classroom" as a service project. You should be able to draw on your organization's strategic funding plan to create a strong sustainability plan.

Evaluation—Foundations require a project evaluation so they can see the measurable impact their funding has on the community. Many people resist conducting an evaluation, put off by the time and money required to collect and analyze data and other information relevant to the project. Do not be intimidated—your evaluation does not have to be at the level of a medical research study. In fact, the evaluation process—with or without statistics—can be critical to the success of the project. See below for a discussion about conducting evaluations to meet foundations' demands and your own organization's needs.

The Ins and Outs of Evaluations

An evaluation can tell you how well your efforts are succeeding, how to fix any flaws in those efforts, and where those efforts could be made more cost effective. The complexity of the evaluation should roughly equal the complexity of the project. More complex programs may call for an outside evaluator, someone who can examine the program more objectively, use her experience to construct surveys and tests, and free your staff to work on the program instead of on the evaluation. If you choose not to hire an independent evaluator, consider hiring a professional to design the evaluation. Ask your local community foundation or university sociology department to recommend an independent evaluator.

Even if your organization cannot afford to hire a consultant, you can still conduct a reliable evaluation. With a little planning, you will be able to conduct a useful and credible evaluation that not only will satisfy the foundation but also provide your organization with the invaluable information it needs for program success.

First, consider the audience and the purpose of the evaluation. Of course, your chief audience will be the foundation, but other interested parties will include your board of directors, other foundations and donors, your executive director, key staff, and volunteers. The evaluation can be useful in

- planning (financial and strategic) by your board of directors

- changing the program to make it more effective

- encouraging more financial support for both the program and your organization

- enhancing public relations through a press release to the media and print materials

To be most effective, the evaluation will likely have two sections, the process evaluation and the outcome evaluation. The process evaluation looks at how the project is conducted. The outcome evaluation looks at the results of the project—specifically, it will show how well the project met the measurable objectives included in the grant proposal. The process evaluation should examine all of the steps laid out in your project management plan. If, for example, the project is an in-school humane education program, you might examine how the schools learn about the program, how volunteers are recruited for the program, and whether the program schedule works well for both the teachers and the volunteers.

Your project management plan will help you identify key players with information critical to the evaluation. (In this example, these may include school principals, teachers, and volunteers.) How do you obtain this information? Generally, your process evaluation may include some or all of the following data-collection methods:

- interviews

- surveys

- tests and other assessment instruments

- review of minutes, reports, or other documents

- focus groups

- case studies

Which methods you use will depend on the purpose of the process evaluation. As you select these, focus not just on what the evaluation will reveal about the current project, but also on how the evaluation can help future projects and programs. If, for example, your organization's short-term goal is to expand its humane education program, an interview with teachers could include not just questions about how they learned about the current program but follow-up questions related to program expansion as well.

The source of the information can also affect selection and application of the method. For example, the evaluator may choose to survey the volunteers anonymously to remove any peer pressure that could result in inaccurate or incomplete responses. In this case, a survey would allow volunteers to respond more honestly than they might in a face-to-face interview.

In an outcome evaluation, the evaluator examines the outputs and outcomes. Outputs are the quantitative results of the program. (In the case of the humane education program, the chief output would be the number of students served.) Outcomes are the qualitative results of the program.

The hypothetical humane education program has two measurable objectives for the project:

- One hundred fifty children in grades one through three at Stevensville Elementary will participate in the humane education program.

- Seventy-five percent of the children will demonstrate gains in their knowledge of the importance of treating all living things with kindness and respect.

The first objective measures an output; the second measures an outcome. It is easy to count how many children were served by the project, but how do you measure gains in knowledge? One option is to test the children. Test their knowledge of humane issues once before the humane education session and test them at the end of the program. Comparing results from the two tests shows how many children improved their scores—and presumably their knowledge. While this evaluation will not pass any scientific validation tests, it should be adequate to meet the requirements of most foundations.

Budget—The budget frequently comes near the end of the grant proposal package, but it should never come last in your priorities. In fact, the budget is often the first thing the reader will review. The program budget is a major factor in the foundation's decision on funding your organization, so make sure the budget reflects a complete and accurate picture of the program. Everything discussed in the narrative should be in the budget, and every cost item in the budget should be in the narrative. Go through the narrative carefully and note all items, activities, and personnel that cost money, even if they are provided as an in-kind expense.

When creating the budget, consider these tips:

- Avoid asking one foundation to fund the entire program. Your research should guide you in how much money to seek from a particular foundation.

- Provide a budget for the entire program; do not just show how the grant will be spent.

- Always include in-kind funds from your organization that will be put toward the program. Some foundations will not allow administrative or indirect costs (such as telephone and photocopying expenses), so consider including those costs in your organization's in-kind contribution. Consider which of these costs might be included as direct costs.

- Determine such expenses as your cost per animal served and per classroom served. These figures provide the foundation with a good idea of the program's cost effectiveness.

- Provide a budget narrative and make sure it explains how you arrived at the costs of each item.

- If you mention staff by name or title in the proposal narrative, list them individually in the budget.

- Proofread the budget carefully and make certain that any costs mentioned in the proposal narrative are the same as those that appear in the budget.

- Have someone else proofread the budget and check your math.

Attachments—Foundations typically request that your proposal includes these attachments:

- determination letter from the IRS showing that your organization has 501(c)(3) status

- audited financial statements and/or your Form 990

- budget for the organization's current fiscal year

- bylaws of the organization

- board of directors list

Don't Say Goodbye

Once you have developed a relationship with a foundation, you want to nurture it carefully. Do not place the foundation on your mailing list unless you know that it wants to receive this information. The program officers are busy people, and they are inundated with mail. Instead, make any mail you send them really count. Invite them to your next gala—but include a personal note. Treat them as individuals, not as names on a mailing list.

If you receive the grant, send a formal thank-you letter signed by your executive director or board chair.

Make careful note of the foundation's reporting requirements. It may want quarterly and final reports of the project's activities. Even if it does not, send the foundation a brief note about any major success the organization has during the funding period. When the project is completed, send the foundation a short report on what was accomplished. If you can provide evaluation results, so much the better. These reports, whether required or not, are key to maintaining a good relationship with the foundation.

If you do not receive funding the first year, do not despair. The first step is to call the foundation. Explain that you understand that it has limited funding but ask if it can make any suggestions for improving your chances in the next year. Then send a polite thank-you note as a follow-up to your conversation. These simple actions can mean the difference between success and failure in future applications, so be certain to follow through no matter what the foundation decided to do about your current proposal.

Try, Try Again

Yes, all this is a lot of hard work for what once seemed like free money for the asking. In a sense, the money is available for the asking—only the asking requires finding the right listeners and getting them to read through your well-thought-out, multiple-page request. So be prepared to spend a lot of time framing that request.

Will the answer be yes? For those organizations that have what it takes—time and a commitment to research projects and prospective grant makers, develop relationships with foundations, create thorough, professional proposals, demonstrate progress, and maintain connections—grants can provide funds for exciting new programs (and even mundane but essential projects). You never know until you try.

Chapter 9

Preparing for Future Gifts: How to Develop a "Planned-Giving" Program

In 2003 National Public Radio received a $200 million bequest from philanthropist Joan Kroc. Sounds like a lot? Wait until you see her bequest to the Salvation Army: $1.5 billion.

True, your organization is unlikely to get such a sizeable bequest in its lifetime. But many animal care organizations receive substantial donations through bequests—assets left to the charity in the donor's will. According to Giving USA *2004 Report* (The Center on Philanthropy at Indiana University 2004a), gifts made through bequests were estimated to be $21.6 billion for 2003 (Figure 9.1), which accounted for 9 percent of total estimated giving and represented an increase of 12.8 percent over the revised estimate of $19.15 billion for 2002. What are you doing to encourage donors and supporters to make these "last gifts" to your organization?

Figure 9.1

Giving by Bequest, 1963–2003 ($ in billions)

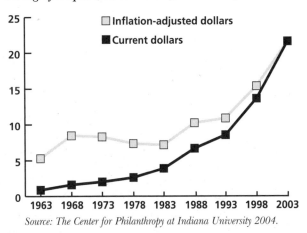

Source: The Center for Philanthropy at Indiana University 2004.

Is It Worth the Effort?

When you go after bequests, you are engaging in a type of fund-raising called "planned giving." Typically, planned giving requires that you do a lot of work now to secure the promise of money you may not see for many years. Why do it?

Planned giving builds long-term organizational viability. Through a successful planned-giving program, your animal care organization can establish an endowment or reserve, fulfill its long-range plans, and establish a cushion for emergencies. Since the average size of a planned gift is $10,000, and the up-front costs are relatively low, your planned-giving program will probably have the lowest fund-raising cost of all of your development functions.

Are You Ready?

Planned-giving programs may not be your most expensive programs to run, but they can be among your most complicated to set up and operate. Remember, with a deferred gift, a donor will not be around to make sure you are using the gift in the manner she requested. You need to demonstrate that your organization is worthy of donors' trust.

Going over these questions can help you decide whether your organization is ready to move ahead:

- Is your organization's work ongoing?

- Is your organization financially solid?

- Do you have a clear vision of where your organization is headed?

- Do you have an active, responsible governing board?

- Do you have sound finances that can be documented with audited financial statements?

- Do you have sufficient staff and access to experts to administer the types of planned gifts you hope to secure? (See planned-gift descriptions in this chapter.)

- Do you have the equipment, software, and technical support required to run your planned-giving program?

- Can you demonstrate evidence of longevity to your prospects?

- Does your organization enjoy a good reputation in your community?

It can take easily five to ten years to see the fruits of your labor. If your organization is struggling to meet its current needs and you are concerned about its solvency, spending a large portion of your time on planned giving probably does not make sense. On the other hand, if your organization has been established for a while, is able to balance its budget, and has a good reputation in the community, then devoting time to develop planned giving will help ensure the long-term strength of your organization.

Planning Today for Tomorrow's Gifts

Planned giving can be as simple as a donor leaving your organization a specific amount of money in his will or as complicated as a "charitable lead trust," a specialized estate planning tool (see Going to the Next Level, below).

A "planned gift" can be either a current or a deferred gift (one that "matures" because of the death of the donor). Current gifts provide immediate support for your organization but require more planning than a typical annual gift. These gifts typically fall under the planned-gift category: real estate (land or the attachments to land); personal property (any other property a person can own, such as cars and jewelry); and appreciated securities (stock that has increased in value since the donor acquired it). When they donate their appreciated property, donors benefit through avoiding capital gains taxes and receiving a tax deduction for fair market value.

The simplest and most common types of planned gifts are arranged through bequests, life insurance, and retirement plans.

Begin with Bequests. Support received from a deferred gift is not realized until the donor is deceased. More than 80 percent of planned gifts are bequests. A donor can choose to leave your organization a specific amount, a percentage of his total estate, or a percentage of his residual estate (the portion remaining after specific bequests are made). Your organization can also be named as a contingent beneficiary to receive all or a portion of the donor's estate if the primary beneficiaries predecease the donor or they no longer exist. Until they die or are no longer mentally capable, donors can change their wills, so bequests are considered revocable gifts.

Learn about Life Insurance. Donors can use their life insurance to support your animal care organization through their estate planning. To do this, the donor names your organization as the initial beneficiary or a contingent beneficiary to receive all or a portion of her life insurance policy. This option is especially useful for donors who have existing policies that no longer serve their original purpose. For example, the donor may have purchased the policy because she wanted the safeguard for her young children. If those children are now self-sufficient adults, the donor could change the beneficiary to your organization and thus leave a legacy for animals. A gift of life insurance, like wills, is revocable until the death of the donor.

The rules differ when a donor buys a new life insurance policy that names your animal care organization as both owner and beneficiary. In this case, the gift is irrevocable. The best way to handle this is for the organization to be the owner of the policy with the insured person paying the value of the premiums to the organization. That way, there are no issues at the death of the insured, and the donor gets a tax deduction every year when she sends the charity a gift to cover the policy.

Rest Easier with Retirement Funds. Another fairly easy way donors can support your organization through estate planning is with their retirement funds. This option offers the donor great tax benefits. If left to someone who is not a spouse, the donor's retirement funds get hit with both income and estate taxes. If instead these funds are left to a nonprofit, both of these taxes are avoided. Here again, donors are free to change the designated beneficiary.

Going to the Next Level

The logistics involved with other types of deferred planned gifts are even more complex than their titles suggest, so consult legal and financial advisors before trying to solicit these "life income gifts," which provide income to the donor for a period of time. (The descriptions below are brief summaries; see Resources for books and web sites that offer comprehensive explanations.)

Gift Annuities. In these contracts between the donor and the charity, the donor agrees to provide the organization a sum of money and, in exchange, the organization promises to make fixed payments to the donor for life. The rate of return on a gift annuity increases as the donor gets older. Gift annuities are irrevocable, but the organization must keep its end of the bargain by making ongoing payments. Gift annuities allow the donor to help his favorite charity, receive steady payments, and enjoy tax benefits. The organization gets to keep a sizeable chunk of the original sum: on average, 50 percent of the original value of a gift annuity remains for use by the nonprofit after the donor's death. Because of the work and expense involved in managing gift annuities, most organizations set a minimum contribution.

Charitable Remainder Trusts. Through these arrangements, donors give the nonprofit organization property in a trust in exchange for an income for life (or a term of years). This income may or may not go to the donor. Charitable remainder trusts may be established through a will to benefit a designated individual. The income can be a set amount (referred to as an annuity trust) or a percentage of the assets of the trust (known as a unitrust). These charitable remainder trusts can be structured to fit the donor's needs and can provide important tax benefits for the donor and her estate. The nonprofit receives the remainder of the irrevocable trust when the last beneficiary dies or the term expires. Because of the work and expense involved in managing these trusts, many organizations set a minimum contribution amount.

Charitable Lead Trusts and Charitable Income Trusts. These trusts are the reverse of the charitable remainder trust. Through charitable lead trusts and charitable income trusts, the income from the trust is provided to the nonprofit for a specified number of years and then reverts to the donor or other named beneficiary. Charitable lead trusts permit transfer of assets at reduced gift and estate tax costs.

Pooled Income Funds. These funds are similar to mutual funds. The donor buys "shares" of the fund and receives an income based on his share of the overall fund. These gifts are irrevocable and can provide a current income tax deduction. Since the nonprofit can sell appreciated assets without paying capital gains tax, a pooled income fund may provide higher income for the donor than the individual currently earns on his assets.

When your organization enters into any of these agreements, it assumes the financial, legal, and ethical responsibility to manage assets for the benefit of your donor. What's more, your organization has to make complicated financial decisions about when and how to spend the money it receives.

Because of the delay in return and the unpredictable nature of planned gifts, many organizations will use these gifts to set up a reserve or an endowment—funds whose principal is invested in perpetuity and the organization uses only the return on the investment. Your board, with help from financial advisors, must decide how and when to use the gifts: will the organization use the bequests for annual needs, or will it set all or some portion aside for reserves? Will this be decided annually or set up beforehand?

Do not earmark bequests routinely to balance the annual budget. When a bequest is added to reserves or endowments, honor the donor by allocating a percentage of his gift to a special project or program. For example, if Mr. Money leaves Small Town SPCA a specific bequest of $500,000, the board could allocate $50,000 to upgrade the deteriorating kennel runs in his honor and put the remaining $450,000 in reserves. Bequests lose their impact when used routinely to supplement basic operation funding or if they disappear into savings.

To operate its planned-giving program, your organization needs professional help. Ask board members, staff, and volunteers to recommend attorneys specializing in estate planning or financial advisors experienced with planned-giving vehicles or contact your local or state bar association and your local planned-giving council for referrals.

Pets in Wills

The community views your organization as an expert in responsible pet ownership, so you can expect some supporters to seek your help on providing for their pets in estate plans. Your organization has a unique role to play here, but be careful not to make promises you can not fulfill.

For example, some animal care organizations have established pet guardianship programs that provide for the ongoing care of their donors' animals. This is an admirable attempt to help people and their pets, and such a program can draw donors to your planned-giving program. But these ventures are resource-intensive, difficult to manage, and full of ethical quandaries. Here are just a few of the questions you will face when planning a pet guardianship program:

- Will you house donors' pets at your facility? If so, how will you provide a high quality of life for an animal indefinitely confined to a cage or kennel?

- How does providing long-term care at your facility fit with your organization's mission and philosophy?

- Can you be responsible for the long-term care of a pet for five, ten, or fifteen years?

- Do you have the necessary space, time, and staff to provide on-site care, run a foster-care service, or find these pets new homes?

- Will operating a pet guardianship program adversely affect any of your other programs or animals in your care?

- How will your organization and the pet owner agree on such complex and emotional issues as providing intensive medical treatment, responding to severe aggression or mental deterioration, and deciding when to euthanize? Who decides—the executive director or a veterinarian?

- What types of animals will you accept? Just cats and dogs? What about snakes or horses?

- Are you prepared to provide care for a variety of animals of differing ages, health conditions, and temperaments?

- How many animals will donors be able to enroll in the program? How will you place pets from multipet households?

- Will you establish a minimum gift level? Will the money be for the animal's care or a general bequest to your organization?

Few animal care organizations are set up to provide long-term or permanent on-site guardianship programs. After all, most organizations already struggle to find the space and resources to care for the endless stream of incoming homeless animals. Even running a temporary guardianship program through foster homes and placement can overwhelm the resources of a small, busy animal care organization.

For most animal care organizations, the best way to help is to encourage donors and the general public to provide for their pets by doing one or more of the following:

- Include their pets in their estate plans by finding a friend or family member willing and able to provide their pets with a permanent home. If they are unable to find a friend or family member to care for their pets, pet owners should discuss other options with their executor or personal representative.

- Create a so-called "side letter" to accompany their wills that specifically provides for their pets. (To have legal legitimacy, the letter needs to be signed, dated before the will, and referenced in the will itself.)

- Check with an estate attorney to find out whether their state allows "pet trusts" to provide funds for the care of the pet for life.

- Maintain information about their pets—name, type, sex, spay/neuter status, age, normal weight, identification information, photo, health history, veterinarian contact, daily routine, preferences, etc.—in their central, accessible files for friends or family members who may end up as the pets' guardians. (Such information can be helpful as well if the animal ends up at the shelter because the executor of the will or the family is unable to find someone to care for the pet.)

For pets-in-wills information that you can share with your supporters, see Resources.

Starting Slowly but Steadily

What type of planned gifts should your organization set its sights on? Start simply. Begin by encouraging your loyal supporters to include your organization in their wills. The National Committee on Planned Giving refers to this as "Phase One: The Bequest and Beneficiary Designation," suggesting that "for many organizations, it may not be necessary, prudent, or affordable to progress beyond this stage of the gift planning process."

Starting simply does not mean you can proceed without a plan. Like most of your fund-raising programs, a planned-giving program requires that you follow certain steps.

Choose your objectives—Review the level of bequest support your organization has received over the past five to ten years and consider where you would like to be in the coming five to ten years. Remember that the planned gifts you solicit this year will likely take a long time to mature. The amount of planned-gift support you want to work toward will influence the amount of staff and board time and financial resources you will need to dedicate to reaching that goal. Consider short-term objectives such as increasing (by a certain annual percentage) the number of supporters who specify that your organization is in their estate plans.

Develop a calendar of activities—Set up deadlines and stick to them. More time-sensitive duties will displace planned-giving activities unless you establish some deadlines for this program. These essential planned-giving activities likely include:

- developing some expertise on your staff or board about planned gifts;

- creating or contracting for basic written materials;

- reviewing your donor base for potential prospects;

- deciding if you want to create a recognition society;

- developing marketing and recognition plans for your program;

- holding training for your board and staff; and

- educating current donors about how to include your organization in their plans.

Establish a budget—Analyze your calendar of activities to estimate the time and financial resources necessary to carry out that plan. Although your budget should cover out-of-pocket consulting and other upfront costs, do not overlook pro bono options. Do you have an estate planning professional on your board or among your volunteers who can assist with the training and development of materials? Can you find a printer to print your materials at no cost or at a reduced rate? At a minimum, your budget should include consulting, training, printing, and recognition activities.

Your board should be involved in this plan every step of the way. Your board members should be the people most committed to the mission of your organization, and they should be willing to demonstrate their devotion by making their own bequests to your animal care organization. This also sends the message to other donors and prospects that those responsible for the organization are committed to its long-term future as well. (For more information on board responsibilities in fund-raising, see chapter 5).

Finding Your Way into Donors' Estates

Start simply, too, when it comes to finding planned-giving prospects. You don't need to drive down Millionaire Lane to find them. Any donor can make a planned gift.

Your best planned-giving prospects are likely to be your longtime, loyal donors—and often your smaller donors. The older donor who has been giving your agency $25 a year for twenty years is an excellent planned-giving prospect. As you delve into your database, concentrate on donors who have demonstrated confidence in the work of your organization. Of course, do not neglect your wealthier, less supportive donors either.

You do not need to start with glossy planned-giving marketing materials to pull in these planned-gift givers. Some easy options include a check-off box in your direct mailings for donors to request information; articles and donor profiles in your shelter newsletter; and informational seminars on general estate planning and including pets in wills. After you have sparked donor interest, do not delay in fulfilling their requests.

When you meet with these donors, listen for clues of their interest in planned giving: "I wish I could do more, but I'm on a fixed income." "I wonder what will happen to my pets when I die?" "I really should start planning for my retirement." These comments can be conversation openers for you to talk about the planned-giving options your organization offers.

Putting It in Writing

As interest grows and the planned-giving program progresses, so will the need for more substantial materials.

As you create a list of planned-giving materials to develop, collect samples from other organizations—and not just from animal care organizations. If you know an estate planning professional willing to help write your planned-giving materials pro bono or at a heavily discounted rate, you are ahead of the game. If not, consider using preprinted materials. Many companies offer off-the-shelf brochures that can be personalized with your organization's logo or, in some cases, customized to fit your needs. See Resources for a list of planned-giving publications.

Tailor your materials and mailings to the targeted audience. For example, a mailing to longtime, loyal donors or to your largest donors might include a testimonial cover letter from someone who has included your organization in her estate planning or a story of a donor whose bequest has helped to change the lives of homeless animals: "$1 Million Donation from Mrs. Greenbacks Builds a Cattery to House Tiny Town Humane Society's Adoption Cats" or "$5,000 from Mr. Dollars Sponsors a Two-Day No-Fee Spay/Neuter Clinic for Residents of Needy Neighborhood."

This mailing should also include your standard planned-giving material and a reply form so donors can request more information or inform you of their decision to include your organization in their estate plans.

Thanking Donors Before You Get the Gift

Most planned gifts come to your organization after the donor's death, which means you will not be able to thank the giver when you get the gift. It is important to plan ways to recognize these donors now, while they are still living. When the person dies and leaves you the bequest, make sure to acknowledge and thank the donor's family members. Not only is this a thoughtful gesture, but it is also a way to bring them into your circle of supporters.

One way you can recognize the donor is through a "legacy society" or "estate planning donor club," which gives you the chance to show your appreciation publicly. Consider mounting a plaque in your shelter engraved with the names of planned-gift givers. Invite them to an annual thank-you event. List them in your annual report of donors. But ask first. Some donors may not feel comfortable talking about their will details or participating in a legacy society; these donors may not even let your organization know of their intent. Do not push these donors—respect their privacy.

Thanking donors amenable to public or private acknowledgment is important for all types of fund-raising. It is the right thing to do, but for planned-giving programs, it is critical for another reason: planned gifts are revocable. Donors can change their minds at any time. Thanking these donors frequently, keeping them abreast of your latest programs and projects, and finding ways to keep them involved in your work can help them appreciate how much their gift means to your organization and the animals it serves.

Chapter 10

Selecting Special Events: How to Run a Winner

Only the hard-hearted dislike watching adorable doggies prance in a dog walk, and the winter holidays just are not the same without "Pets with Santa" photos. Such special event fund-raisers, favored by both animal care organizations and pet-loving communities, are great fun and an important part of your development program.

But the fun does not always translate into big money. The enticing events draw people and their wallets, but they can draw away your time and resources as well. If you are not careful, you may end up spending more to produce the event than you raise from people attending it.

Do not let that caveat cause you to cross special events off your list of fund-raisers. When done well, special events can play a key role in an organization's overall fund-raising and outreach program.

What Good Are They?

Well-planned and -executed special events can be much more than moneymakers. Plan your event to take advantage of these extra opportunities:

Draw new donors. Your goal is to bring in new money, not redirect money that is already coming into your agency. Consider whether the proposed event will bring in new donors, raise more money from existing donors, or tap into funding sources you are not currently reaching. If not, ask whether the cost in financial and human resources is worth what you will gain from the event.

Attract media attention. Animal care organizations have a special advantage with the media: animals make for popular visuals. Proper event planning should include a comprehensive media plan that gives the media—especially print and television—the opportunity for pictures with cuddly creatures. Events typically attract one-time or short-term media attention, so you will still need to maintain media focus between events.

Increase public awareness of your organization. Your organization depends on name recognition and community awareness for funding and other support. Special events can give you this, which may seem reason enough for holding them. But do not confuse special events with community outreach events. Special events can provide excellent exposure, but they are designed to raise money. Community outreach events, on the other hand, attempt to generate publicity and to raise the level of community awareness of your organization or a specific program. For example, holding an open house to celebrate your organization's anniversary or the opening of a new shelter can be a great vehicle for bringing people to your shelter or for media publicity, but it may not be a good vehicle to raise money.

Expand your support network. Special events offer great chances to enlist new volunteers and bring in new donors. Many people prefer to volunteer for an annual event rather than make an ongoing commitment, but this does not mean they are not committed to your organization. With proper cultivation, training, recognition, and communication, they can be wonderful community ambassadors. Make sure all volunteers working at your special event understand your organization's mission, programs, and services. This information will provide these volunteers with a greater appreciation of and enthusiasm for your organization, which they can share in turn with event participants and their friends and family.

Consider, too, how your proposed special event may appeal to new donors. Different events draw different people, so think about the desired audience. For example, some events—a celebrity comedy show, for example—are themselves the draw, meaning that many people come for the show no matter what organization benefits. These events can generate money but may not generate loyal donors. On the other hand, people parading with their pooches in your organization's annual dog walk are dog lovers who appreciate your work for animals.

Appeal to the business community. Take the opportunity to show businesses how contributing to your special event will benefit their bottom line. A printing company may be willing to print the invitations in exchange for its name and logo on them. You can offer your underwriters or sponsors a chance to have their logo or ad in an event program and provide contributors with complimentary event tickets. Mind your manners and send a proper thank you to contributors—this may even gain you their future assistance. (See Get Down to Business Sponsors, below, to learn more about securing sponsorships.)

Educate board members and volunteers. Special events can be a good introduction to fund-raising for your board members and volunteers. Many people who are uncomfortable with other types of fund-raising prefer special events, which offer something concrete in exchange for the ticket price or registration fee. By asking their family, friends, and co-workers to support an event, these board members and volunteers begin to see who supports the work of your agency.

Not Everything Is Special

Special events offer advantages that other forms of fund-raising cannot, but these events also offer some disadvantages that their counterparts do not. For one thing, attention is often drawn to the event itself, not to the mission of your organization. Many attendees go to enjoy the event, not to show commitment to your organization. To shift attention back onto your organization, keep the focus of your events on animal issues. A fun, animal-oriented event can acquaint the uninitiated with the great work of your organization. Capitalize on the opportunity to cultivate new donors and follow up with those who may provide greater support—potential major donors and those with valuable business and community contacts.

Another drawback is that many special events are one-price-fits-all, offering minimal opportunity for varying donation levels. While you can design events with different ticket prices or levels of registration, generally people will select their own level of participation. In these situations it is awkward if not impossible to encourage larger gifts. So how do you make sure that your current major donors do not start supporting your organization at a lower level? When possible, secure the donors' annual commitment before sending them an invitation to the event. If the timing does not work, explain to donors beforehand that the price of the event is considered separate from their usual support.

In special events, the cost per dollar raised can range from "losing money" to 20 percent or less. (Most agencies look for a 50 percent or lower cost.) Since the cost per dollar raised can be higher than other forms of fund-raising, be careful that you are not redirecting current donors.

Fund-Raising for Animal Care Organizations

Let's say that Mr. and Mrs. Royce, who typically make an annual $200 donation to Sunny City Humane Society, receive an invitation to a $200/couple dinner-dance for that organization. After paying event expenses, the organization nets $75 instead of the usual $200 from that donor.

How do you avoid spending too much money producing a special event? How do you avoid hosting a special event that draws attendees who care more about the attraction than your organization? Start by selecting the right special event.

Pick Me, Pick Me!

Congratulations! After five minutes of brainstorming, your group came up with a bunch of ideas for great events with cute, catchy names. Now the planning can begin, right?

Slow down. You need to spend a lot more time analyzing each idea, no matter how irresistible the event theme or name. The success of your special events program depends on selecting the right events. Before selecting one, ask these questions:

Will the event help us meet our goals?

What are your fund-raising goals (both gross and net revenue)? How much do you want this event to raise? What are your marketing goals? What kinds of publicity or name recognition would you like to generate?

If you hope to generate $25,000 in revenue, an event that will draw 150 people at $25 a ticket is not going to work for you (and no, you will not be able to solicit enough in sponsorships to make up the difference). As you examine these fund-raising goals, consider how much you can spend on that event—you have to spend money to make money.

Do you need the event to generate publicity and exposure for your organization? If so, a golf tournament—unless it includes Tiger Woods—is not the best choice. If you do not have access to celebrities (certain to lure the media), plan a unique event with a special twist and, of course, irresistible photo opportunities. Some creative events with these visual lures have included puppy reunions, a mascot adoptee leading your walk, ribbon-chewing openings, and pet/owner look-a-like contests. (See Spread the News, below, for more about media exposure and developing a media plan.)

Will the event help you raise awareness about important issues and your organization's role? If this is your top goal, it may be best to plan a community outreach event instead of a special event fund-raiser. But even if generating awareness falls below your goal of generating money, take advantage of exposure opportunities. For example, decide on two to three facts that you want to impart to all attendees. Then sneak that information into all event promotions, publications distributed at the event, and follow-up material.

Does the event compromise our mission?

When selecting special events, have your organization's mission statement and policies close by. If you have a policy promoting vegetarianism, you should think twice about holding a fund-raiser at a popular downtown steak house. Deciding whether a special event meshes with your mission is not always easy. For example, if your organization opposes circuses and other events that exploit performing animals, is it okay to hold a Halloween event in which pets are paraded around in costumes? You may rule in favor of this special event—after all, these are beloved companion animals, not neglected wild animals or circus captives. Still, it is critical that you weigh the implications of each proposed event, however innocent it may be on its surface.

Go through this process before accepting a contribution or sponsorship for your special event. Partnering with a business implies that you endorse that business, so do not let a tempting donation cause you to compromise your organization's values or reputation. Make sure everyone in your organization understands your mission and knows which businesses are "off limits." You do not want to be placed in the awkward position of turning down a contribution from a business approached by a well-meaning but ignorant board member (see chapter 4 for more information on ethics).

Who is our audience?

What people do you want to attend your special event? "The general public" is too vague an answer, so be more specific. Are you targeting dog owners who like to participate in activities with their pets? Do you want to draw young families? Single young adults? Women in their thirties and forties? Residents of a particular geographic area? Your choice of audience will influence the type of event you select and its scheduling and cost. For example, if you want to draw young families with children, a Wednesday evening (school night) event probably will not work. To help you select the right event and the right schedule for your target audience, try preliminary field testing. Run some ideas by people who represent that audience to help you plan for their needs and expectations.

Do we have people power?

You may have financial resources, but do you have human resources? Special events are labor-intensive—you need lots of people with specialized skills to pull off a successful event. For example, a benefit dinner and silent auction require that people—your board members and volunteers—sell enough tables to achieve your revenue goals.

Planning alone takes a lot of time and a lot of people. Even if you have a strong volunteer force, understand the trade-off. Time spent organizing an event takes away time from other valuable programs. Make sure you use your volunteers wisely. That time spent by a well-connected board member to create flawless centerpieces could be better spent soliciting her business associates for major gifts. In this case, time really is money.

After working through all these issues, you have concluded that the event will meet your organization's fund-raising goals, suit its mission, attract the desired audience, draw appropriate media exposure, and receive the necessary volunteer support. Good work. Now the real planning can begin.

Timing Is Everything

Before you pencil the event into your organization's calendar, make sure you examine the community's calendar. School is out and the weather is fine, but the second Saturday in June may not be the best time for your annual dog walk event if other nonprofits are holding pledge walk/runs the same weekend. Are you considering a black-tie event? First find out whether and when other organizations have scheduled similar dinners. Businesses and individuals often have ties to several different community organizations and may not take part in similar functions held the same evening or too close together.

Consider your staff and volunteer schedules and your entire fund-raising calendar. Even though two events or activities may be months apart, both may require a lot of work at the same time. Can your staff, board and volunteers do it all?

Even if they can, and even if they are fast workers, plan your event several months, not weeks, in advance. You must allow enough time for sponsors to make decisions and to add their support for your event to their budgets. The desired room or location may require booking months or a year in advance, and designing and printing promotional materials and event invitations takes time. None of this can be thrown together at the last minute.

As you plan the event, create a timeline that works back from the date of the event and allows enough time for all of the required tasks (see the sample timeline in appendix D.10). Make sure your plans include both a step-by-step outline of all procedures involved in the event and instructions covering rules, equipment, clean-up, and other necessary details (see sample standard operating procedures for the Distraction Dash in appendix D.12).

Spend Money to Make Money

Your budget should include revenue and expenses. To plan your budget, examine all the ways you will try to generate revenue. Revenue should include ticket sales, registration fees, table sales, ad booklet sales, sponsorships, silent or live auction pledges, vendor sales, and individual donations and pledges. Then analyze each of these revenue goals to determine what it will take to reach them. How much money will you have to raise first to pay for the special event designed to bring in funds later? Your budget must detail not just the expected revenue, but also the necessary up-front costs. (For ideas, see the sample budget in appendix D.9.)

Make It Legal

Before you go any further, make sure you get the necessary permits and licenses for your event location and activities. Ask the site owner about necessary permits (typically detailed in the contract). If you are using a park or other public location, ask the overseeing government agency which permits you will need. For an event at your shelter, check your building capacity for safety issues (exits in case of fire or other emergency). Serving alcohol or food? First find out whether you need any special permits. Regulations may differ for events selling alcohol or food versus for those events providing free refreshments. Sellers may need a license.

You will also need to make sure you comply with IRS requirements (see chapter 4).

Someone Has to Do It

You have created a detailed "to-do" list in your timeline, but do you know who will tackle the tasks? Do you have enough skilled volunteers to take these on, or will staff, volunteers, and board members work together? Jobs range from soliciting sponsorships to stuffing registration packets. You may find it helpful to develop job descriptions for those responsible for chairing the event, soliciting sponsorships, coordinating the auction, handling ticket sales, arranging for rentals, planning the program, and coordinating setup and cleanup. (The people holding these positions may form your event steering committee.) In the job descriptions, clearly state your expectations for each position, highlight the deadlines, and detail the chain of command (who reports to whom).

If your organization plans a high-profile special event, consider asking a board member to chair the event. The chair must be enthusiastic about the event, possess the necessary leadership skills, be willing to delegate tasks to others, and contribute to the success of the event. Local celebrities or other notable people can be named as honorary chairs even if they don't have time to do any of the work. Sometimes just the "big name" is enough to add credibility and draw interest. You also may consider naming a shelter animal as an honorary dog or cat chair.

Even if few volunteers are required in the planning phase, more helping hands will be needed the day of the event. So as you envision the event unfolding, picture where volunteers will be stationed and what they will be doing. How many people do you need at registration or at T-shirt pickup? How many volunteers do you need for event setup and dismantling? How many volunteer "tour guides" are needed to help guests navigate the event? If pets are on site, do you need volunteers to watch the guests' dogs while they use the restrooms or get food or bid on auction items?

Whether they are working at the special event or planning it, all volunteers need orientation and training to help them fulfill their responsibilities. Everyone involved should understand the organization's mission and basic policies, the special event structure and purpose, and his role in making that event a success. Make sure volunteers working at the event itself receive advance training so they understand exactly what they will be doing. Events can be crowded and busy, and you do not want your volunteers to feel flustered or frustrated. To help the event run smoothly, provide the volunteer with a follow-up letter reminding the person of his responsibilities. (See appendix D.11 for an example.)

Spread the News

No matter how exciting your event, people will not attend if they do not know about it. How you spread the news depends partly on your target audience, so plan your marketing strategy accordingly. And be creative—people are inundated with information these days, so design your material to catch their attention. Here are ways to spread the word:

Save-the-date cards. These notices encourage people to mark the date of your event on their calendars, so recipients may be more likely to open the invitation when it arrives.

Invitations/brochures. Mailing an event invitation or informational brochure helps highlight your event and initiate response. (The type—invitation or brochure—depends on the type of event.)

Media sponsors. Media sponsorship can include public service announcements or free advertising, talent provided for the event, links from their web sites to yours, and live broadcasts from the event. As you develop media sponsors, you'll likely interact with the community outreach and advertising departments. Ask them to connect you to the right people in editorial departments to generate stories about your event. To help spark the interest of print and TV media sponsors, be sure to highlight photo opportunities in your proposals. (After all this hard work developing media relations, don't neglect them during the rest of the year. Maintaining close relationships with the media can help your organization in all it does, not just special events.) Consider developing a formal sponsorship kit for both local businesses and media that lists the year's sponsorship opportunities.

Shelter newsletter. Use your organization's newsletter to inform donors of upcoming events and how to sign up. You want to lure new donors to the event, but you also want to provide current donors with opportunities to help you and encourage support from their friends.

Community and business newsletters. These publications often seek stories that interest their residents or employees. A short piece about your "Paws 'n Claws" benefit dinner may be just what they are looking for. When you approach the newsletter staff, ask if they would be willing to donate ad space to help you publicize your event.

Notices in utility bills. Ask your utility company if it can help sponsor your event by including a promotional flier advertising it in their utility bills.

Notices in thank-you letters. Add a note or a separate notice to your thank-you letters to remind donors of any upcoming special events.

Posters. Distribute posters advertising your event around your facility and throughout your community.

Signs. Yard signs, street banners, and restaurant tabletop signs are inexpensive ways to get the word out about your event.

The web. More and more people are using the web to learn about community. Do not neglect the Internet's power as a marketing tool:

- **Information on web site**—Be sure to include information about your event on your organization's web site. Highlight the event with a banner on your home page that sends visitors to an events page for details.

- **Internet newsletter**—If you e-mail electronic versions of your newsletter or include them on your web site, make sure you highlight your event. Start with a "teaser" several months out and mention the event regularly in subsequent issues. As the event draws closer, make your event ads and stories more prominent.

- **Online registration**—If your organization has this capability, consider adding online event registration. Many people prefer this method to mail-in or in-person registration.

- **Online pledging**—If your event requires participants to raise pledges, see whether you can help participants set up web sites to facilitate the process. For example, participants could send out their own e-mails asking friends and family to sponsor them and provide links that allow these donors to make their pledges via a web site.

These are just a few of the many marketing ideas available to you—be creative. Whatever methods you choose, remember to encourage advance ticket purchases and registrations as much as possible. With advance purchases, you will have a better idea of how many people to expect. For outside events subject to unpredictable weather, advance registration and ticket purchases help protect against low turnout.

Let Us Entertain You

When you first came up with the idea for your event, the facts probably were a little vague: some dinner with some "big name" and maybe a silent auction. Now it is time to get down to the details. If you are planning a dinner, are you going to provide entertainment? What will the program for the evening look like? Who is speaking, when, and about what? If you are planning a walk, what time will registration start? When will the walk start? What happens at the end of the walk?

This is also the time to think about whether you want to include a celebrity entertainer or speaker. Celebrities can add visibility to an event, attract media attention, and draw participants, but many will charge at least a percentage of their normal appearance fee even if they support animal welfare. Consider, too, that your organization may need to pay for travel and hotel for both the celebrity and his staff. That is why it is essential that you find out about any out-of-pocket expenses and special requirements before arranging for celebrity entertainment. A similar rule applies to musical entertainment. Find out what the band expects your organization to supply and determine audiovisual equipment requirements. It is worth the time and cost to have an attorney review your contact with a celebrity before you sign it.

Plan for a Rainy Day

As you plan your event, make contingency plans in case something goes wrong. What will you do if a freak hailstorm is forecast for your fabulous outdoor event? Who will save the day if your guest of honor gets sick? What happens if you over- or undersell the venue? How will the audience hear if the audiovisual equipment fails? Just as you plan for what you want to happen during the event, make sure you plan ahead so you can handle the unexpected.

Special Considerations for First-time Events

First-time events present special challenges. You do not know exactly what to plan for or how many people to expect. As you plan this event, make sure selected activities, desired target audience, and revenue goals match up.

Do not reinvent the wheel. Search your community, web sites, or publications like *Animal Sheltering* magazine to learn about similar events held by other organizations. Do not be shy—ask these agencies for advice about what worked and what did not. Some organizations may even provide you with their written procedures, task lists, calendars, and other helpful tools.

Do You Need Professional Help?

If you are overwhelmed with special event planning, consider pulling in the professionals. Here are some sources to explore:

Party planners. An event consultant or party planner may be just the person to help you through a first-time event or add new life to an existing event. Before hiring a consultant, know exactly what you need, what the consultant offers, and how much the service will cost. Find the right planner for your party. A party planner who focuses on events for wealthy individuals or for businesses may have great ideas but may not understand the special needs of nonprofit organizations. If you hire a professional, watch that person carefully so you can learn how to plan future events on your own.

Outside organizations. What happens if a company representative calls with an offer to carry out a benefit event for your organization? As tempting as this sounds, do not agree to anything before you learn the details. What exactly will the business provide? What does it expect from your organization? How will the event be staffed? How will funds be raised, and what portion will go to your organization? How will people be invited? What other organizations, if any, will benefit from the event? Both parties must understand and agree on who does what and who gets what. If the company can organize the event but expects you to sell all tickets, can you fulfill your end of the bargain? Do you have a large enough donor and volunteer base to sell enough tickets to make the event worthwhile? It may be better to decline the offer if you cannot meet expectations than to participate in an unsuccessful event.

Event software. If your organization does a lot of special events, explore computer software designed to help in planning and tracking them. Start by finding out if your development software's vendor offers a special events package that works with your existing software.

Get Down to Business Sponsors

Celebrities. Bands. Fancy dinners. How on earth are you going to pay for all this? Most special events require your organization to fork over a lot of money before getting any proceeds. Business sponsorships can help, and here's what to do:

Go prospecting. Your list of potential prospects should include businesses with connections to your board members and volunteers; businesses that have supported your organization; vendors your organization uses; and businesses that want to reach your intended audience.

As you develop your list, find out who makes the decisions and how to reach these key contacts. Keep track of your contacts, the requested support level, the sponsored event, and the responses.

It is all in the approach. First you will need to show potential sponsors what they get out of the deal and what contribution is expected (e.g., cash, product, or in-kind services).

Try approaching potential sponsors at the beginning of the year with a sponsorship kit for all of your organization's special events. Doing this one time, all at once, not only shows sponsors that you respect their time, but it also helps you use your time more effectively.

If your first approach gains you a "go away," do not give up. Even a rejection can help you improve your chances next time. Ask the business why it is not able to sponsor your event, and consider what you might offer or do differently next year that would gain you their support.

Play up the benefits. Most businesses participate in event sponsorship because they see a benefit for their companies. Sure, they may want to help your organization as well, but this is likely a secondary consideration. As you develop your sponsorship levels, be specific about the benefits the company will receive. What advertising or marketing opportunities can you offer? Consider what will appeal to different sponsors. For your "Pooch Prance" walk-a-thon, for example, maybe you can offer a car dealer the opportunity to have one of its vehicles be the lead car around the course. Pitching and planning marketing opportunities requires a lot of preparation on your part. If your event provides an ad book, how will you determine ad size and dollar amount for each sponsorship level? If you have a newspaper sponsor, can you include the business sponsors' names or logos in the ad? Will you include the sponsor's name or logo in your event invitation, registration form, newsletter, web site, and posters? Can you fulfill sponsors' requests to distribute their products to event attendees? Are you willing to let the business do a direct marketing mailing to attendees?

Make sure you can—and should—deliver before promising specific marketing opportunities to potential sponsors.

Present a proper proposal. Make your proposal professional and concise. Include marketing information about the event: number of attendees and their demographics (such as age ranges, gender, and income levels); ways you plan to promote the event; and the link between the demographics of your attendees and the businesses' target audience. If you are approaching a pet supply store in your community, point out that your event will be reaching "X number of women in pet-owning households between the ages of twenty-five and fifty." (For more information on demographics, see appendix A.)

Proposals for first-time events typically contain assumptions and estimates about the target audience. Proposals for subsequent events, however, should provide solid information on attendees to help you sell future sponsorships.

If possible, make an appointment to present your proposal in person. If this does not work, mail the proposal and contact the recipient within a week to answer any questions and find out the next step. If you are told, "We'll call you," do not sit by the phone forever; call the business if you do not hear back.

Do not rush them. Allow plenty of time for the business to make a decision and for you to follow up. It may take several calls or visits to get an answer. Be patient—remember, businesses do not consider event sponsorship a priority in the way you do. Many larger businesses set aside a certain amount of money each year for marketing and event sponsorship. Pay attention to their timelines and budgeting schedules.

Make it multiyear. As you develop these relationships, consider negotiating multiyear sponsorships—especially for your larger or more established events. Some proposals may contain a set rate for each year's event; this may work well for table sponsors at an annual dinner if you plan to increase ticket prices each year. Other proposals may request gradual increases of funding levels; consider this type for the title sponsorship of an annual event that is experiencing significant growth in participants and exposure.

Business involvement. Are there ways for the employees or customers of the sponsoring business to participate in your event—as volunteers, a corporate team, or attendees at the sponsor's table? Help businesses understand that such involvement can translate into positive press— almost free advertising—when people see the company's commitment to the community and its support of an important cause.

On-site perks. Consider whether and how sponsors can garner attention at the event. Can you place banners around your event site? Can sponsors have booths? Can you print a registration form, invitation, or admission ticket that includes the sponsor's name or logo? Will the master of ceremonies announce the sponsorship? Should you award a plaque to special sponsors?

Heap on the praise. You cannot thank your sponsors enough. Mail a formal thank-you note immediately after a business agrees to sponsor your event and a second letter after the event (be sure to include event results). Also send copies of any materials (such as brochures, invitations, and T-shirts) that displayed the sponsor's name or logo. As an added touch, consider sending sponsors of one event complimentary tickets for another. Or invite sponsors to a thank-you event at your facility. Think of ways to stay in touch with your sponsors throughout the year, taking care not to pester them with sponsorship requests.

Calling It a Day

Your event is over. Everyone had a great time and rewarded your organization with much-needed funds. It is tempting to congratulate yourselves and move on to the next project. However, if you want your future events to enjoy the same success, you have a bit more work to do.

Show your appreciation. Thank everyone involved. Make sure to send thank-you letters to your sponsors, volunteers, participants, and hosts or celebrities telling them how much you appreciate their support and reporting the results of the event. Depending on the type of event, small thank-you gifts for your sponsors, committee, or hosts or celebrity may be appropriate. These gifts can be presented before, during, or after the event.

Be careful not to take your employees, staff, and board members for granted. It is important to thank everyone—not just those who worked directly on the event but also those who helped keep the rest of your activities running.

Take a look back. Evaluating the results of your event will help you identify what was successful and what you would like to change for the next event. Begin by comparing the actual revenue and expenses with the budget you created. Then look at the original goals you had for the event. Did the event meet them?

Gather together all who helped plan or who participated in your event for a debriefing. Review what went well and what did not. This is the time to find ways to improve, not to assign blame for things that went wrong.

Try to get feedback from the outside, too, by sending a follow-up survey to a random sample of participants. Sometimes what you learn may surprise you. For example, what the participants liked and did not like may differ from the views of your volunteer and staff "insiders."

Keep in touch. Event follow-up can be a cultivation tool for building stronger relationships. Do not end things with the thank yous: stay in touch with everyone who was involved in your event. First, add all of the participants' names to your mailing list. Then sit down with several knowledgeable volunteers and board members to review the participant list for people who may be major donor prospects for your organization. Keep the number of prospects manageable, but do not miss this opportunity to gather information about your participants and supporters (see chapter 6).

Use event follow-up to plan your next steps with sponsors, too. Are there other ways they can be involved with your organization? Are there ways you can assist their business? Future connection will depend on the business and your organization's programs and services. Be creative. For example, invite some sponsors to your next event or present a seminar for some of their employees.

Also review the list of the event's volunteers. Whom can you ask to assume a larger role in next year's event? Planning for future events also means doing some leadership planning among your volunteers.

Gear up for next year. It is never too soon to begin planning next year's event. Even as you plan your current event, jot down ideas that can help improve next year's. Combine those ideas with the suggestions that come out of the evaluation process and begin to create your plan for next year's winning event.

To learn more about how animal care organizations structure their event timelines, event budgets, and the events themselves, see the examples in appendix D.9–D.12.

Chapter 11

Carrying Out Capital Campaigns: How to Bring in Big Money for a Big Project

Need a new sheltering facility? Want to create a state-of-the-art mobile spay/neuter clinic? Projects costing hundreds of thousands of dollars will not happen with money raised from bake sales, no matter how delicious the brownies. To raise this much money, you need to explore a capital campaign.

A capital campaign is an intensive, organized fund-raising effort to raise money for specific capital needs or projects, executed within a specific period (usually over one or more years). It requires careful study, planning, and identification of major potential donors, and it lays the groundwork for involvement of new volunteers and donors.

It's No Small Affair

The capital campaign is the largest fund-raising campaign your animal care organization can take on. Organizations launch capital campaigns for specific, restricted, large-scale projects such as facility construction, renovations, equipment purchase, and endowment development. (Using money received through a bequest or generous corporate, foundation, or personal donation for such a project does not constitute a capital campaign.)

A capital campaign differs from standard fund-raising methods. The annual fund, for example, uses a variety of solicitation techniques to support operations and solicits gifts from current income payable within the fiscal year. A capital campaign, on the other hand, focuses on personal solicitations and relies on pledges of cash or assets payable over three to five years. Only a small portion of your constituent base will be major prospects for a capital campaign.

You can expect to spend between eight months and several years in preparation before making the first solicitation for your capital campaign.

If your organization finds itself in a perpetual struggle to secure resources for even basic operations, then you are not ready to undertake a capital campaign. An organization must be financially stable to initiate such a campaign, which entails significant up-front planning, time, and resources.

No Leadership Means No Campaign

A capital campaign is the responsibility of the board, and the board's giving becomes the cornerstone for the campaign. If you do not have a strong, committed board, you cannot have a capital campaign.

The board's first responsibility is to determine if the need for funds is justified and whether a campaign is required. If that decision is yes, then the board and volunteer leadership must support the campaign for it to succeed. Board members must be willing to participate in solicitations within their means and circles of influence.

A capital campaign requires extraordinary teamwork. (For more information about board leadership, see chapter 5.)

For information on hiring a consultant for your capital campaign, see Hiring a Capital Campaign or Direct-Mail Consultant, below.

Step One: Get a Plan, Fran

The first step is the planning phase, during which you establish a statement of preliminary goals and a plan of action. During this phase, you will develop your case statement, conduct a feasibility study, plan your pre-campaign actions, and enlist leadership.

1. *Capital campaign plan.* You cannot begin the capital campaign until you get clear and agreed-on policies and guidelines detailing how the campaign will run and how funds will be handled. This written plan must cover all aspects of campaign operations, including:

   - campaign policies and guidelines

   - fund-raising strategies

   - role of the leadership task force, staff, and other volunteers

   - communication plan

   - campaign budget

   - timeline of the campaign and pledge period

   - procedure for recording pledges

   - procedure for depositing gifts

   - rules on recording other gifts, such as annual fund and bequests

   - guidelines for accepting non-cash gifts

   - authorization for assignment and transfer of securities

   - recognition opportunities and criteria

   - procedure for final campaign wrap-up and audit (including creating an audit committee)

2. *The case statement.* The case statement, which spells out the reason and rationale for the campaign, serves as the basis for all solicitations, whether from individuals, corporations, or foundations.

   - Your case statement will include the organization's mission statement, history, need for service, services provided, current reports (for both animals and financials), and staff listing (with recognition and accreditation). Include the board, advisory board, and task force lists, revenue sources

Fund-Raising for Animal Care Organizations

and allocation charts, growth charts, and successes. Paint a picture of the need with projected financials, a drawing of your proposed building or photo of equipment desired, and a gift-range table (see Step Four: Collect Pledges, below).

■ This information should be bound and printed for distribution, but it does not need to be slick and glossy. Your publications should reflect your cost-conscious organization and the economic climate in your community. The format should be reader-friendly, containing charts, graphs, photos, drawings, and bulleted text. You do not want potential contributors to struggle through paragraphs to understand your case.

3. *Leadership planning task force.* Create a short-term leadership planning task force to help you develop a case for financial support. The task force should contain fifteen to twenty community leaders with proven leadership experience in other organizations. These leaders should understand community animal issues and should support the organization's mission to provide comprehensive animal programs. The task force will:

■ review the organization plans and set priorities for future development

■ review pre-program and campaign strategy and recommend refinements

■ review the case statement draft and recommend necessary changes

■ review prospect lists and make suggestions for major prospects and potential hosts from various markets

■ assist in host recruitment for pre-program community public awareness meetings

■ advise board and staff on major prospect strategy

■ assist in introductions and cultivation

The task force should not be disbanded before it delivers endorsed organization plans and priorities for development; a draft case statement to communicate to various major prospects, seeking involvement and ownership; a strategy for preparing and implementing a capital campaign; a prospect list for possible major gifts after the pre-campaign preparations; and lists of priority major prospects and volunteers for enlistments and solicitation. When its work is done, you should be well on your way to launching a capital campaign.

4. *Feasibility study.* Your feasibility study tests the concept of the campaign and gathers data for the campaign plan. Why not conduct the feasibility study first, before devoting so much work to creating a campaign plan? To accurately determine whether a campaign is feasible, first you must analyze a comprehensive plan. The purpose of the feasibility study is to determine whether that plan, created by the task force, is realistic.

The feasibility study involves confidential interviews of a broad spectrum of community leaders, donors, and others. Interview questions commonly include:

■ What is your attitude toward the ABC Humane Society?

■ What is your perception of the Society's professional and volunteer leadership?

■ What is your feeling concerning the proposed plans presented in the case statement?

■ What type of campaign would be appropriate in XYZ County for the ABC Humane Society?

■ Are you willing to give to this organization?

■ Are you willing to work to raise the money?

■ Is the goal achievable?

Ideally, the feasibility study should be conducted by a professional who can provide the confidentiality, objectivity, and experience necessary to determine the likelihood of the campaign's success. These feasibility study results are reported to the board of directors, whose members are charged with determining whether and how to proceed.

What should you do if the feasibility study results indicate that your organization is not ready to conduct a capital campaign? Your team should analyze the study carefully to determine what your organization lacks. Perhaps the study will reveal that your organization is not well known in the community, that the public does not know enough about your program, that the organization is not meeting the needs of the community or the animals, or that the public holds unfavorable opinions (e.g., views the organization as unprofessional). Try not to be offended or defensive about the study results. Instead, view the findings as an opportunity to fix critical flaws that could have resulted in an expensive and disappointing campaign. Then, after going back to the basics and resolving the underlying problems, conduct a new feasibility study before launching your campaign.

5. *Pre-campaign planning.* With your up-to-date strategic plan in hand, case statement draft ready for testing, and internal prospects identified, you are ready for the next step: the internal audit. Many people cringe at the word "audit," but in this case it simply means that you will need to closely examine:

Organization planning—What is the internal consensus about your organization's mission and direction? You need to identify program plans for the next five to ten years and understand their long-range funding implications.

Board leadership—How involved and knowledgeable are the people serving on your board? Evaluate board membership and the nomination/recruitment process, review committee structures and board relationships, assess board members' involvement and effectiveness in fund-raising, and review their role in the capital campaign planning process.

Administration and finance—Do you know what everyone does and where everything is? Analyze staff size, experience, capabilities, and organization. Take a look at how goals and objectives are created and their outcomes evaluated. Assess record-keeping systems, gift receipts and acknowledgment procedures, fund-raising programs, prospect research and management, donor cultivation and recognition programs, and support materials and programs. Note, too, that if you are building a new shelter, you need to budget for additional ongoing operating expenses that may increase significantly.

Donor base—How many donors do you have? Who are they? How much do they have and how much can they give? Use your development software to help you analyze these how, who, what, why, when questions: number of donors; levels of giving for campaign; constituency size, location, and age distribution; trends among similar organizations; and past and current campaign obligations.

Volunteer structure and involvement—How much do you really know about your volunteers? Examine how your volunteer system is organized, how many volunteers you have, how they are involved in fund-raising, and how staff supervise and support them.

Public and donor relations—How do people view your organization? Is it well known? To improve strategies for reaching your target audiences, review your public relations efforts, including advertising, media relations programs, publications, community-based programs, and special outreach efforts.

Leadership enlistment—Volunteer enlistment must begin at the core of the campaign, with recruitment of an energetic, well-respected campaign chair. This can be someone who participated in the leadership task force or who was identified through that process.

Volunteers are essential to a successful capital campaign. They are involved by option, not obligation, meaning that they believe in your organization and support the campaign. Skilled, committed, passionate volunteers can recruit other helpers, who recruit other helpers, who recruit other helpers. This domino effect builds your volunteer campaign team.

Step Two: Cut to Cultivation

With all the work you have already put into planning the capital campaign, you are probably anxious for some serious payoff. But first you will need to find potential payers. That is where the second phase of your capital campaign comes in: the cultivation phase.

During this development phase, you will pique prospective contributors' interest by exposing them to your campaign. Here you will market the case among key constituencies—those closest to your organization, including your board of directors, other inside groups (such as volunteers and trainers), the top one or two prospective donors, and even close friends in the media. The development phase also includes testing the reaction of prospective donors and volunteers; responding to questions (before solicitation); building ownership of the plan; developing print and audiovisual materials; securing media attention (for the organization, not the campaign); and positioning and possibly securing early leadership gifts.

Let's Meet Over Breakfast

You will have to learn to like—or at least tolerate—meetings during this phase. Start by holding a series of small "awareness meetings" for friends of your organization and community leaders to outline your plans for a major fund-raising program. Your goal is to gather guidance as you launch this comprehensive resource development planning process.

Find a host with a sincere interest in improving the quality of life in your community. Event venues may vary—breakfasts, luncheons, afternoon meetings, happy hours, or dinners—but the hosts' roles will not. Make sure you select a host who can carry out these sequential tasks competently:

- Meet with staff to review their roles and create an invitation list for the awareness meeting.

- Personally invite the desired guests.

- Follow these phone calls with letters of confirmation (prepared by the organization).

- Preside at the awareness event with an agenda and script (prepared by the organization) and provide appropriate snacks/refreshments.

- Send each participant a letter of appreciation (prepared by the organization).

The host also does some detective work during these get-togethers as she searches for potential leaders and givers among the guests. Follow-up responsibility then shifts to the organization.

Structuring a Successful Awareness Meeting

Your organization's capital campaign awareness meetings cannot be casual, thrown-together gatherings near the water cooler. These are formal affairs of around fifteen to thirty important people who can contribute to the success of your campaign. Hold the meetings in quiet, private settings such as a country club, private meeting room, or residence where you can interact with everyone.

Keep the meetings short, no more than two hours. To keep the meetings running smoothly, follow these agenda guidelines:

- During the reception period, the host meets, greets, and introduces guests to your organization's representatives and other guests.

- After asking guests to be seated and thanking them for attending, the host briefly reviews the meeting agenda, expresses her faith in the organization's plans, and introduces the speaker.

- The speaker from the organization reviews the case statement, shows any drawings or models of the project, and entertains guests' questions and comments.

- When the speaker has finished, the host briefly endorses the organization's plans, encourages guests to provide guidance, and urges those interesting in hosting future meetings to call the organization's representative.

■ As the meeting concludes, the host thanks the guests for attending and officially closes the event.

This process is a great way to grow awareness in your community, build leadership, and identify potential donors. During these meetings, watch guests' reactions to help you fine-tune your case statement and strategies.

Step Three: Ask and You Shall Receive

Now you are ready for "the ask." The solicitation phase should begin at the top and from within the organization. First ask your organization's board of directors, staff, other inside groups, and one or two top prospective donors. These "gifts of confidence" provide credibility for the campaign and sanction an organization to begin widespread solicitation.

In a capital campaign, gifts are solicited in sequence, beginning with those with the highest giving potential and moving to those evaluated at the next lower levels. The first phase is the "quiet phase," during which the organization's "family" is solicited for lead gifts. The goals of the quiet phase are:

■ obtaining 100 percent board participation

■ securing the top one or two gifts needed to ensure the campaign's success

■ reaching approximately 40 percent to 50 percent of the campaign goal before public announcement

Half of the money collected for the campaign will be received in four to six gifts. If you cannot achieve this first goal, then you should either postpone your capital campaign until you can or lower your expectations. The gift-range table, sometimes called the scale of giving, represents average gift levels needed to complete the campaign. Your top-rated prospects will be in the leadership division, and prospects evaluated at the middle of the gift-range chart will be in the major-gifts division.

Think of the chart as a road map to guide you, not as a recipe for the exact mix of gifts you must acquire. A capital campaign goal must be reached on paper before it can be achieved in real life. See Step Four: Collect Pledges, below, for a sample gift-range table from a successful capital campaign to build a new animal shelter.

When your organization does reach that 40 percent to 50 percent goal, you are ready to quit the quiet phase and go public. Taking the campaign into the larger community requires selling your organization and the capital campaign to prospects outside your inner circle of known supporters.

You will need to promote not just your organization but also the need to build that new state-of-the-art animal shelter. Spread the word about your capital campaign through such vehicles as a campaign newsletter, web site link, community awareness events, and press announcements. In addition to reaching out to broader audiences, you will need to focus on one-on-one meetings with prospects.

This requires volunteers with inside knowledge about your organization, its mission, and the proposed project; confidence and people skills; and training in how to approach, engage, and ask prospects to support your capital campaign. (For guidance on how to approach prospects and prepare for the "big ask," review chapter 6.)

As the organization moves into this active solicitation phase, each volunteer will call on an average of five prospects. Help campaign volunteers analyze the donor list to understand each prospect's giving potential and likely gift range (e.g., $100,000 and above; $25,000–$99,999;

$10,000–$24,999; and under $10,000). This process sets the priority sequence for cultivation and solicitation. Always start with likely donors (those who have given before) and work your way down to those who have never given to your animal care organization.

Soliciting gifts for your capital campaign is a lot more challenging than selling T-shirts at your annual dog walk. Your organization's campaign director must provide comprehensive training for all volunteers and unite prospects with the right volunteers. The campaign director must be an effective cheerleader and support person to keep your volunteers' spirits up and help them stick to deadlines.

The time frame for this solicitation may be two months (or longer if you need to cultivate more prospects). But do not let this phase be open-ended: create deadlines and schedule status meetings to instill the sense of urgency necessary to propel your campaign.

Step Four: Collect Pledges

The final step of your capital campaign is the pledge and fulfillment phase. But do not expect to collect all of that promised money overnight. Generally, a three- to five-year collection period is built into the campaign plan. It is not unusual for that time frame to extend even a year or two beyond the pledge period.

Although you may not see capital campaign funds right away, that does not mean you should hold off showing your appreciation to contributors. Make sure you thank your donors appropriately and keep them informed of the campaign's progress. (For more information on ways to thank and involve your supporters, see chapters 6 and 7.)

The Gift-Range Table

The gift-range table, sometimes called the scale of giving, represents average gift levels needed to complete the campaign. As stated earlier your top-rated prospects will be in the leadership division, and prospects evaluated at the middle of the gift-range chart will be in the major-gifts division.

Think of the chart as a road map to guide you, not as a recipe of the exact mix of gifts you must acquire. A capital campaign goal must be reached on paper before it can be achieved in real life. Here is a sample gift-range table from a successful capital campaign to build a new animal shelter (Table 11.1).

Table 11.1

Gift Range   *$3,500,000 Campaign*

Number of Gifts	Range	Cumulative Total
1–2	$500,000–1,000,000	$1,000,000
3–4	250,000–500,000	750,000
5–6	100,000–250,000	500,000
7–9	50,000–100,000	350,000
10–15	25,000–50,000	250,000
16–25	10,000–25,000	160,000
26–35	5,000–10,000	130,000
36–100	3,000–5,000	108,000
101–300	1,000–3,000	101,000
Many	Under 1,000	151,000

Hiring a Capital Campaign or Direct-Mail Consultant

Do you need a capital campaign or direct-mail consultant? Most organizations need these consultants unless they have someone on staff experienced in running a capital campaign or managing direct mail. These consultants offer specialized skills and specific services when current staff lacks the experience or time to provide them.

Before selecting a consultant, interview several different fund-raising consulting firms. There are many good firms, but it is important to find the one that best meets your organization's needs.

Remember, too, that although you may be hiring a consulting firm, you will be working primarily with an individual assigned to your capital campaign or direct-mail project. Too many organizations hire firms that send them people who have never run a capital campaign or managed direct mail. That is why it is critical not only to get the person's resume but also to ask probing questions. Asking the firm the list of suggested questions below can help you find the best person for the job.

- Describe your consulting firm, its philosophy, length of time in business in the area, and staff available for consulting.

- How many current clients do you have? Can we call all of your current and former clients for references?

- Have any of your campaigns been for humane organizations?

- What is the largest campaign you have managed? What is the smallest campaign you have managed?

- Who will be directly supervising the on-site campaign director? How often will we see this person?

- Please outline your work/staff plan.

- What is your fee? Many fund-raisers subscribe to a code of ethics that prohibits them from being paid based on a percentage of funds raised. Work with a fund-raiser that bases its fee on the amount of time spent working with you—for a capital campaign—or on the amount and type of mail managed—for direct mail—and not on a percentage of funds raised. (For more information on ethical fund-raising, visit the Association of Fundraising Professionals at *www.afpnet.org* or call 800-666-FUND.)

Suggested questions to ask the person who will be working with you directly:

- How many campaigns have you run? (The consultant should have run the actual campaigns rather than just worked on them.)

- How long have you been with your current firm?

- How long have you worked in fund-raising?

- Can we call all of your former clients (with whom you have worked personally) for references?

■ What professional fund-raising organizations are you a member of?

■ Outline your previous fund-raising experience and describe the professional training you have received.

Suggested questions to ask a potential capital-campaign consultant:

■ How often will you be on-site?

■ Where do you volunteer? Where do you contribute? (It is important to hire a campaign director who knows what it feels like to be a volunteer and donor.)

■ How long have you been in the area? (Knowledge of the local funding community is critical. It is also important to have a consultant who does not have to fly home every weekend.)

■ What are your personal areas of fund-raising expertise? What is your experience in securing major gifts? What experience do you have with planned giving? Prospect research? Direct mail? Writing grant proposals?

■ What is the largest gift that you personally have secured?

Chapter 12

Wandering the Web: How to Take Advantage of Online Fund-Raising

Let's assume that you are a local animal care organization that gets the majority of its funding from residents. Does it make sense to spend time exploring online fund-raising that reaches beyond your borders? If you are still a bit skeptical about the well-touted "powers of the Internet," you are in good company. But that does not necessarily mean you are right. Both for-profit and nonprofit organizations—even smaller ones—have a lot to gain from a presence on the Internet. Here are just a few numbers to show you why:

- An estimated 185 million people in the United States use the Internet.

- *The Computer Industry Almanac* projects that 1.85 billion people worldwide will use the Internet by 2006.

- The Pew Internet Project reports that 60 percent of Americans are online and 72 million people have made a purchase online. Such online purchasing is growing rapidly as people discover that it is safe, fast, and reliable.

- Donations of more than $1,000 brought in 8.3 percent of all dollars raised online in 2003, according to a survey of 3,151 fund-raising campaigns.

The interest in the Internet is already there—you just need to find creative ways to take advantage of it. Through your organization's electronic mail, web site, and other online avenues, you have the potential to reach more animal lovers and potential donors than you can with other fund-raising methods. And with the vast information sources available on the Internet—from informal fund-raising newsgroups to national nonprofit assistance sites, your organization can trade tips with other humane groups and research the latest information on foundations.

It is relatively inexpensive to set up a web site and electronic mail system that can reach people not just in your hometown but throughout the world. Imagine if you had to pay printing and postage costs to connect to all of the people—potential supporters—who could receive your e-mails and visit your web site. This low cost and high potential opens up new opportunities for innovative fund-raisers.

There is a "but": while online resources can answer some of your fund-raising dreams, the web can turn into a nightmare if you expect too much or prepare too little. For example, e-mailed notes to donors can never replace the all-important face-to-face visit. Launching an online fund-raiser—such as an online auction or gift store—without first addressing new ethical and legal challenges can get you into trouble. Your animal care organization can and should explore how the Internet can help your fund-raising goals. You just need to adopt the careful research and planning that you practice in all of your other successful fund-raising strategies.

Checking Your E-mail

Even if you still prefer using a pen to using a mouse and think *amazon.com* has something to do with a rainforest, you most likely use e-mail, if only occasionally. It is growing increasingly more difficult to do business or even communicate with friends without access to electronic mail.

E-mail has become a popular, and even essential, tool for fund-raising—and for good reason: E-mail can be a quick, cost-saving way of communicating with donors and supporters in your community. Michael Gilbert of the Nonprofit Online News (*www.nonprofitnews.org*) recommends these "Three Rules of E-mail" to help nonprofit organizations:

- Resources spent on e-mail strategies are more valuable than the same resources spent on web strategies.

- A web site built around an e-mail strategy is more valuable than a web site that is built around itself.

- E-mail-oriented thinking will yield better strategic thinking overall.

Here are just a few of the ways you can take advantage of electronic mail to reach your supporters and potential donors:

- electronic newsletter

- emergency requests

- thank-you notes

- special event reminders

- project/program status updates

- volunteer opportunities

- animal-related community news

The true power of the Internet for fund-raising, says Gilbert, is the power of personal communication combined with the power of scale. While web sites serve an important purpose, they are passive and cannot actively raise funds for your organization. E-mail, on the other hand, is proactive and promotes person-to-person communication. People read most of their e-mail messages, while favorite bookmarked web sites can be forgotten quickly. So instead of waiting for people to visit your web site, develop an effective e-mail plan that steers people to a stronger relationship with the organization.

Before you begin sending e-mails to people in your community, take some time to educate yourself about a key concept known as "permission-based marketing." If you have or use a computer, then you know that "spam," or unsolicited junk e-mail, upsets people for many reasons: the most often cited one is that people do not want to be bombarded with e-mails they did not ask for.

How do you know if someone wants to read an e-mail from your organization? You will only know if that person has given you permission to send him e-mails. Do not send an e-mail newsletter, fund request, or other electronic communication to anyone who has not opted in to receive them, and honor any requests to remove e-mail addresses from your list.

The good news is that getting such permission can happen at the same time you first get the e-mail address. After all, to send e-mails, you need to begin collecting e-mail addresses from people in your community. So any time you ask for e-mail addresses, such as in your direct-mail pieces or on your web site, be sure to include opt-in language such as, "Would you like to keep in touch with us via e-mail? Please provide your e-mail address." If they give you their address, you then have their permission to send them e-mail communications.

Finally, once you have someone's e-mail address, do not go overboard by sending that person e-mails too frequently. And be sure to keep your messages concise, consistent, personable, and professional. For an example of a professional e-newsletter, see appendix D.15.

Waking Up Your Web Site

Of course, adopting a good e-mail strategy does not mean you should shun the web. An effective web site remains a critical way to self-promote, educate, and fund-raise. A hastily produced, unprofessional site, on the other hand, can backfire. Devote the time and resources necessary to produce the kind of web site that reflects your organization. Your web site does not have to be flashy—in fact, it should avoid those cluttering extras such as how-do-you-turn-this-off background music and dance-across-the-page cat graphics, which serve only to annoy and confuse many visitors. To produce an innovative yet professional web site, get professional help. Seek a web design company that does pro bono work, or try finding a volunteer with this expertise (try *www.volunteermatch.org*).

Make sure that visitors to your web site feel at home and can find what they want. If your visitors are inundated with confusing graphics and cannot figure out immediately how to donate, they are likely to leave the site and not return. Create user-friendly menus with clear, simple options that take visitors quickly where they want to go—such as to your mission statement, board of directors list, planned-giving overview, or calendar of events. Since most visitors are not searching for your planned-giving page, include links to this page (and others you want them to see) or the one that gets the most traffic—such as "animals available" photos.

How does this kind of well-designed, user-friendly site help your organization? A well-managed web site can:

- tell visitors what your organization is and what it does

- (literally) show visitors how your organization helps animals (online photos of adorable animals helped by your organization prove that "a picture is worth a thousand words")

- enable visitors to print donation forms or, better yet, donate online

- highlight your "wish list" for in-kind donations (such as towels, food bowls, newspapers, dog collars, cat litter, etc.)

- introduce your board, staff, and volunteers

- promote volunteer opportunities and other ways to become involved

- provide an audience for your online newsletter and other online outreach publications

- encourage visitors to sign up for more information

The best web site in the world, however, will not do your organization any good if no one visits it. Here is how to make sure you get a lot of traffic to your web site:

■ Develop a clear online identity by producing a distinct brand and succinct description.

■ Network with local businesses—especially animal-related ones—and ask them to provide links to your web site on their own sites. Links from media outlets in your community can drive traffic to your site as well.

■ Make sure that your city government's web site includes your organization's name, contact information, brief description, and web site link.

■ Register your web site with search engines and online directories (check out *www.trafficmagnet.net* and *www.bCentral.com*).

■ Visit *www.selfpromotion.com* for more information on getting your web site noticed.

Electronic mail and a web site do not replace traditional direct mail; in fact, these methods can complement each other. For example, in the hard-copy newsletter that profiles an abused, malnourished dog that came to your shelter, you could say, "For an update on Scruffy's condition, check our web site." This way the reader can find the latest photos and updated information about this and other animals, programs, special events, and services via your web site and e-mailed updates.

How Would You Like to Pay for That?

Many nonprofit organizations make it easy for their web site visitors to make a donation or purchase items on the spot with a credit card. But many people avoid making online payments because they are concerned about security breaches or identify theft. Here are some ways to make people more comfortable donating on your web site:

■ Make sure your donors' information is secure. Talk with your bank to see if it offers online credit card processing.

■ Look into online processing centers, such as *donate.net*, that can connect your site's users to secure servers that take donations for organizations.

■ Consider other payment options, such as *paypal.com*'s online payment services.

■ State clearly on your web site how your site protects users' personal and financial information.

Do not bully your visitors into making online donations. Provide alternatives so all of your potential donors feel comfortable donating to your organization. In addition to secure online payment options, provide an online form that donors can print, fill out, and mail to you. For example, donors can fill out and "snail mail" (via the U.S. Postal Service) an online form in which they agree to have $5 or more charged to their credit cards each month. Also be sure to have the traditional donation form available for donors who want to write a single, one-time check.

To encourage your web site visitors to participate online, provide opportunities that make their lives easier. For example, enable your visitors to register online for events, camps, and obedience classes.

Moving Fund-Raisers Online

If you learn the technical basics, you will be surprised how easily some of your traditional offline fund-raisers can be adapted for online use. For example, many animal care organizations are discovering that moving auctions online can draw a new and larger audience to the bidding battle, and this can translate to larger funds for your organization.

Like many animal care organizations, the Humane Society of Pagosa Springs in Colorado raises money through sales of its thrift store items. But it made more money on certain items when the organization decided to auction off the more valuable donated items on the online auction site eBay. From its first venture into the world of online auctions, the shelter sold nearly $50,000 in a two-year period. Costs are minimal because eBay and similar online auction sites take only a small percentage of the final sale, and the buyer pays shipping charges.

Many animal care organizations also have created online marketplaces that donors can access through the organization's web site. These web-based gift stores allow visitors to purchase such basics as T-shirts emblazoned with your organization's logo and spay/neuter bumper stickers with a few clicks of the mouse and quick online payment. Some organizations process and fill these orders internally, while others team up with online businesses to handle online purchases. Visitors to the Dumb Friends League's online gift shop, for example, are connected to an online "store" powered by *Cafepress.com*.

Cheaper, but Not Free

Handling fund-raising activities online can be less expensive and less time-consuming than many traditional methods. But you will still have to devote money, people, and time to planning, developing, and maintaining an online presence.

For example, you will need skilled individuals— employees or volunteers—to send out e-mails and respond to incoming e-mails. And you will need someone to update and manage your web site. The same holds true for online auctions and online stores, which can be labor-intensive and will require an employee or volunteer with the time and commitment necessary to monitor and fulfill orders.

You also will need to make room in your budget for establishing online fund-raising. You may need to hire a web site development consultant, purchase a "domain name" to secure a web site address, and invest in a digital camera for photographing items you hope to sell through an online auction or an online marketplace. Depending on your resources and your online development plans, you may want to consider working with companies, such as cMarket (*www.cmarket.com*), that help nonprofits conduct online auctions.

Raising funds online also requires that you devote the time needed to integrate your online activities with your other fund-raising methods. For example, your capital campaign status and goals should be highlighted on your web site. And your snail-mail direct-mail pieces should invite people to visit your web site and ask for their e-mail addresses. Make sure that those involved in other fund-raisers work closely with those charged with updating the web site and sending out e-mail updates to supporters.

Before launching any online venture, make sure your organization can comply with the new and varied legal requirements. For example, if your web site asks for donations and can be accessed by residents of other states or even countries, they may view your organization as operating and soliciting funds there. To find out whether and how to register in other states, work with an attorney experienced in these new and confusing Internet legal issues. She can guide your organization in complying with other jurisdictions' requirements and can suggest language for your web site to protect your organization. (For more information on ethical responsibilities, see Principles of the E-Donor Bill of Rights, below, and chapter 4.)

Byte-size Appreciation

Online fund-raising is expanding rapidly, offering innovative nonprofits seemingly limitless opportunities for success. That success depends, however, on viewing the Internet not just as a way to solicit but also as a way to cultivate and maintain relationships with donors. Your donors want to see where their funds are being spent, and you can use the Internet to show them. E-mail supporters with program and project updates and success stories. Provide a prominent place on your web site to highlight what you have been able to accomplish through donor support. And use the Internet, through e-mail and even your web site, to thank donors—even if you have already delivered a snail-mail or verbal thank you. As you progress in the high-tech, impersonal ease of Internet communication, do not forget to add the human touch to all of your online fund-raising activities.

For more information about online fund-raising, see Resources.

The Ten Rules of e-Philanthropy that Every Nonprofit Must Know
(from the ePhilanthropy Foundation)

Rule #1: Don't become invisible. If you build it, they won't just come. Building an online brand is just as important and just as difficult as building an off-line brand.

Rule #2: It takes know-how and vision. Your organization's web site is a marketing and fund-raising tool, not a technology tool. Fund-raisers and marketers need to be driving the content, not the web developer.

Rule #3: It's all about the donor. Put the donor first! Know your contributors, let them get to know you.

Rule #4: Keep savvy donors; stay fresh and current. Make online giving enjoyable and easy. Give the donor options. Use the latest technology. Show your donor how his funds are being used.

Rule #5: Integrate into everything you do. Your web site alone will do nothing. Every activity you have should drive traffic to your site.

Rule #6: Don't trade your mission for a shopping mall. Many nonprofit web sites fail to emphasize mission, instead turning themselves into online shopping malls, without even knowing why.

Rule #7: Ethics, privacy and security are not buzzwords. Many donors are just now deciding to make their first online contribution. They will expect that your organization maintains the highest standards of ethics, privacy, and security.

Rule #8: It takes the Internet to build a community. Many nonprofits (particularly smaller ones) lack the resources to communicate effectively. The Internet offers the opportunity to cost effectively build a community of supporters.

Rule #9: Success online means being targeted. The web site alone is not enough. You must target your audience and drive their attention to the wealth of information and services offered by your web site. Permission must be sought before you begin direct communication via the Internet.

Rule #10: ePhilanthropy is more than just e-money. ePhilanthropy is a tool to be used in your fund-raising strategy. It should not be viewed as quick money. There are no short cuts to building effective relationships. But the Internet will enhance your efforts.

Principles of the E-Donor Bill of Rights

The Association of Fundraising Professionals' E-Donor Bill of Rights, a work in progress, seeks to address new concerns and challenges arising from Internet charitable giving. These principles relate to the AFP's original "Donor Bill of Rights" (see chapter 4) but provide specific guidance to address the emerging ethical issues surrounding the new world of online giving:

- To be clearly and immediately informed of the organization's name, identity, nonprofit or for-profit status, its mission, and purpose when first accessing the organization's website.

- To have easy and clear access to alternative contact information other than through the website or email.

- To be assured that all third-party logos, trademarks, trustmarks and other identifying, sponsoring, and/or endorsing symbols displayed on the website are accurate, justified, up-to-date, and clearly explained.

- To be informed of whether or not a contribution entitles the donor to a tax deduction, and of all limits on such deduction based on applicable laws.

- To be assured that all online transactions and contributions occur through a safe, private, and secure system that protects the donor's personal information.

- To be clearly informed if a contribution goes directly to the intended charity, or is held by or transferred through a third party.

- To have easy and clear access to an organization's privacy policy posted on its website and be clearly and unambiguously informed about what information an organization is gathering about the donor and how that information will be used.

- To be clearly informed of opportunities to opt out of data lists that are sold, shared, rented, or transferred to other organizations.

- To not receive unsolicited communications or solicitations unless the donor has "opted in" to receive such materials.

Literature Cited

Alliance for Nonprofit Management. n.d. Frequently asked questions: How can we do a competitive analysis? *www.allianceonline.org/FAQ/strategic_planning/how_can_we_do_competitive.faq.*

American Association of Fund Raising Counsel, Association for Healthcare Philanthropy, Association of Fundraising Professionals, and the Council for Advancement and Support of Education. n.d. Donor bill of rights. *http://www.afpnet.org/tier3_cd.cfm?folder_id=898&content_item_id=9988.*

American Pet Products Manufacturers Association (APPMA). 2003–2004. National pet owners survey. Greenwich, Conn.: APPMA.

American Veterinary Medicine Association (AVMA). 2002. *U.S. pet ownership and demographics sourcebook.* Schaumburg, Ill.: AVMA.

Association of Fundraising Professionals. n.d. Standards of professional practice. *www.afpnet.org/tier3_print.cfm?folder_id=897&content_item_id=1068.*

———. 2004. *State of fund-raising: 2003 Report.*

BoardSource. n.d. Nonprofit essentials: What is a conflict of interest? *www.boardsource.org/FullAnswer.asp?ID=89.*

———. n.d. Board essentials: What are the responsibilities of individual board members? *www.boardsource.org/FullAnswer.asp?ID=102.*

———. 2002. Board members and personal contributions. *boardsource.org/TopicPaper.asp?ID=71.*

The Center on Philanthropy at Indiana University. 2004a. Comparison of reported success of techniques: December 2001 to December 2004. Glenview, Ill.: American Association of Fund Raising Council Trust for Philanthropy.

———. 2004b. *Giving USA, A publication of the Giving USA Foundation.* Glenview, Ill.: American Association of Fund Raising Council Trust for Philanthropy.

Clancy, E.A., and A.N. Rowan. 2003. Companion animal demographics in the United States: A historical perspective. In *The state of the animals II: 2003*, ed. D.J. Salem and A.N. Rowan, 9–26. Washington, D.C.: Humane Society Press.

DeMartinis, R. n.d. Starting a fundraising program: Where is the money? *About.com: http://nonprofit.about.com/od/fundraising/a/starting.htm.*

Fischer, M. 2000. *Ethical decision making in fund raising.* New York: John Wiley & Sons, Inc.

Independent Sector. 2001. *Giving and volunteering in the United States.* Washington, D.C.: Independent Sector. *www.IndependentSector.org.*

Internal Revenue Service. n.d. Unrelated business income tax—General rules. *www.irs.gov/charities/article/O,,id=96104,00.html.*

Jensen, M. 1999. Information technology at a crossroads: Open-source computer programming. *The Chronicle of Higher Education*, October 29.

Society of Animal Welfare Administrators. 2003. *Survey.* Denver: Mountain States Employers Council, Inc.

The Foundation Center. 2004. *Foundation giving trends.* New York: The Foundation Center.

The Foundation Center's Statistical Information Service (*www.fdncenter.org/fc_stats*). 2004. New York: The Foundation Center.

Vertis. 2003. Customer focus: Direct marketing.
In *Direct mail response figures rise
significantly: Vertis study reveals good
news for direct marketers with the
results of its 2003 customer focus:
Direct marketing study.*
http://www.vertisinc.com/about/viewNews.asp?id=81.
———. 2004. Customer focus 2003: Nonprofit.
In *Two-thirds of the nation plan to make
a non-monetary contribution: New Vertis
study reveals the habits and motivations
of nonprofit contributions.*
www.vertisinc.com/about/viewNews.asp?id=92.

About the Contributors

JUDITH A. CALHOUN, CAWA, (chapters 9 and 10) is vice president of development/community relations for the Dumb Friends League in Denver, Colorado. She oversees all fund-raising and community outreach for the League, including direct mail, special events, foundation and corporate fund-raising, special promotions, major gifts, planned giving, media, marketing, publications, and humane education. Before coming to the League in 1998, she served for five years as director of development for the Peninsula Humane Society in California.

VINCENT F. CONNELLY (chapter 7) is president, Connelly & Associates Fund-raising LLC. A fund-raising professional since 1985, he has directed comprehensive capital campaigns for local and national clients. He is an active board member and a past president of the Association of Fundraising Professionals (Maryland chapter), and he was selected as one of the "Top 40 Under 40" by the *Baltimore Business Journal* in 2002.

JULIE MILLER DOWLING (chapter 12) is a California-based freelance writer. She is a former editor for The HSUS's *Animal Sheltering* magazine and a current HSUS consultant. She has written many articles on animal care issues and is the author of the forthcoming manual *How to Form a Humane Organization*.

CARYN GINSBERG (chapter 2) is co-founder of Priority Ventures Group. She helps animal-protection organizations get better results through strategic planning, marketing, and measurement. She has consulted with organizations, including The HSUS, the ASPCA, and the Spay-Neuter Assistance Program (SNAP). She teaches for Humane Society University and has taught marketing strategy and management for Johns Hopkins University. She also serves on the board of directors of the International Institute for Humane Education.

KAREN MEDICUS (chapters 1, 3, 5, 6, 11) is director of Imagine Humane (a project of the American Society for the Prevention of Cruelty to Animals and PETsMART Charities). She is a Certified Fund Raising Executive (CFRE) with more than twenty-five years of experience in the animal care and protection field. Her varied experiences have included cleaning kennels at a humane society in Maryland, investigating animal cruelty, serving as a major-gifts officer, and leading a humane organization as executive director.

continued...

M. Christie Smith (chapter 4) has been executive director, Potter League for Animals, in Newport, Rhode Island, for more than twenty-two years. Her direct supervisory responsibilities include special events, annual campaigns, capital campaigns, major donors, and planned giving, and her special interests encompass accounting, audits, and IRS requirements. She is a member of The HSUS's National Companion Animals Advisory Group and serves as a consultant for the HSUS Animal Services Consultation program.

Alice Tracy, Ph.D. (chapter 8), is director, Foundation Relations, for The HSUS. She has a highly successful track record in writing grant proposals for both federal government and private foundation funding. She has raised more than $8 million during her career, and her grant proposals have been ranked in the top two or three of hundreds received. She holds a doctorate in English literature from the University of Maryland. For many years she has served as a volunteer and fund-raiser for local animal organizations.

Evaluating Your Community and Organization

Obtaining objective, measurable data will help you spot trends that affect your organization's operations and enable it to deliver the best programs to meet needs and justify continuing financial support. As you assess your community by collecting data on the population you serve, you may discover:

- an increasing number of senior citizens, suggesting more demand for assistance with animal care when people are temporarily disabled and presenting an opportunity to increase planned giving

- growth in ethnic groups, requiring you to adapt your outreach to a different language or culture

- high incidence of neglect or cruelty cases in certain neighborhoods, warranting the allocation of additional resources

Keep in mind the phrase, "What what/So what/Now what," to get the most from data:

- What information do you need?

- What do the data say?

- So what does that mean for the needs of your community and the role of your shelter?

- Now what are you going to do as a result of what you know?

Revealing Who's Who in Your Town

Here are some of the factors you will want to explore to understand your community's population and describe it to funders:

- total population

- age distribution

- income

- ethnic groups

- households

- home ownership

- education

- employment

- marital status

(Be sure to look at information across multiple years so that you can see changes.)

As you gather data, do not overlook free resources. For example, the U.S. government provides census data and information from the American Community survey at *www.factfinder.census.gov*, and *www.easidemographics.com* offers easy-to-use reports. Your local library, planning commission, economic development board, tourism council, and real estate agents can also provide (or refer you to sources for) local population statistics. These groups can help you understand the business community to identify potential sponsors or partners.

Discovering Animal Demographics

In addition to understanding the human population, you will want to zero in on animal-specific information. Unfortunately, the census does not track data on companion animals. Surveys by the American Veterinary Medicine Association (2002) and the American Pet Products Manufacturers Association (2003–2004) estimate that 36 percent to 39 percent of households with animals have dogs and 31 percent to 34 percent have cats. Rates differ dramatically by state, however; for example, 21 percent of Massachusetts households care for dogs versus 50 percent of West Virginia households. You can also incorporate data provided by Clancy and Rowan (2003).

The HSUS's State of the Animals series of monographs (at *humanesocietypress.org*), "State of the American Pet" (*www.purina.com/institute/survey.asp*), and the National Council on Pet Population Study and Policy (*www.petpopulation.org*) provide statistics on issues such as estimated euthanasia rates, reasons for relinquishment, and acquisition sources. Analyzing these numbers can guide your planning, programs, and fund-raising.

Counting Your Community's Furry Blessings

Knowing how many animals are in your area can help your organization plan for the future.

When it comes to obtaining grants, planning outreach programs, and preparing for possible disasters, animal care professionals know that sometimes it is all in the numbers. Foundations, donors, and elected officials usually want to see statistics and hard data supporting requests for more funding.

One figure that often seems difficult to estimate, however, is the total number of owned animals in your community. Even if you have a handle on the number of licensed animals, there will still be a high percentage of people who do not register their pets.

The HSUS's recently published *Disaster Planning Manual* (2100 L Street, N.W., Washington, D.C.) contains advice for those who want to help animals in their community to stand up and be counted. It offers a formula that is by no means exact, but rather is based on national averages. It does not account for potential variables among regions, states, and communities. If, for example, you live in a densely populated suburban area with a large number of apartments and full-time workers, cats may be the pet of choice for many more people with limited time and space. On the other hand, a suburban area with mostly housing developments may be home to a higher number of dog lovers.

Keep such variables in mind so you can make necessary adjustments when using this formula. For the purposes of explanation, we will use the fictional example of Anytown, a community with 100,000 households.

Step 1. Find out the number of households in your community; the local emergency management or property appraiser's office should be able to help with this. In our Anytown example, the number of households is 100,000.

Percentage of U.S. Households Owning a Pet*

Dogs 39

Cats 34

Birds 6

Number of Pets per Household*

Dogs 1.6

Cats 2.2

Birds 2.6

Source: The American Pet Products Manufacturers Association's 2003–2004 National Pet Owners Survey.

Step 2. Using the figures in the table in Step 1, determine how many households in the community own dogs, how many own cats, and how many own birds. You can arrive at this number by multiplying the number of households in your community by the percentage of people who own each species nationally. Here is what the math would look like in a community of 100,000 households:

- 100,000 households in Anytown x 0.39 (percentage of dog owners nationally) = 39,000 dog-owning households in Anytown

- 100,000 households in Anytown x 0.34 (percentage of cat owners nationally) = 34,000 cat-owning households in Anytown

- 100,000 households in Anytown x 0.06 (percentage of bird owners nationally) = 6,000 bird-owning households in Anytown

Step 3. Multiply the numbers you arrived at in Step 2 by the average number of each species owned per household.

- 39,000 dog-owning households in Anytown x 1.6 (percentage of dogs owned per household nationally) = 62,400 dogs in Anytown

- 34,000 cat-owning households in Anytown x 2.2 (percentage of cats owned per household nationally) = 74,800 cats in Anytown

- 6,000 bird-owning households in Anytown x 2.6 (percentage of birds owned per household nationally) = 15,600 pet birds in Anytown

Now Anytown has rough estimates of the number of dogs, cats, and birds in its community. You can also apply this formula to other species, using national statistics for reptile or small-animal ownership.

(Note that there are regional and local differences in the number of households with pets. Typically, cities have lower rates of pet-caring households than do suburbs and rural areas. In fact, you may see as much as a twofold difference from one region to another. However, even a rough estimate is better than none, and it is not difficult to do a quick survey if you really want more accurate estimates.)

Nabbing Numbers from Inside

Often your organization already has the most useful data. What type of information do you have that would yield insight into the status and prognosis for your animal care organization? Statistics on incoming and outgoing animals by type and reason can help you detect changes in your service area, quantify the scope and success of your operations, and identify issues that could necessitate action and attract support. For example, if your shelter is experiencing challenges with incoming feral cats, did you see that coming before you were overwhelmed?

Incoming and Outgoing Animals by Type and Reason

Example: For dogs, cats, and other animals separately and combined:

Starting and Incoming, by Source

In shelter and foster care at beginning of month

Incoming:
- strays
- owner relinquished
- transfers from other shelters
- seized animals

Outgoing, by Disposition and Ending

In shelter and foster care at end of month

Outgoing:
- redeemed by owner
- adopted
- euthanized
- died
- transferred to other shelters
- animals on hand at the end of the month

Mine your records for other revealing numbers and information, such as:

- program activity levels—such as for spay/neuter, wellness services, micro-chipping, cruelty cases, animal training, and humane education

- where your clients come from (by zip code) and how they heard about your shelter

- where most animals come from (by zip code)

- feedback on clients' experience with your organization (such as from satisfaction surveys)

- your member database and donor history

- statistics kept on licenses, dogfighting citations, or other animal-related activities

Your community and funders seek measurable outcomes from your work. These data will help you and your management team establish a baseline, set objectives, measure performance, and report on results. Visit *www.petpopulation.org* to learn more about why you should track these statistics and to obtain detailed recommendations on what to collect.

Knowing Your Strengths and Weaknesses

Collecting and analyzing these data gives you a better understanding of what is happening in your organization and in your community. Perhaps you have observed that your organization is well prepared to meet the need for more subsidized spay/neuter services. Or maybe you have discovered that there are too few investigators to handle the growth in cruelty cases.

Identifying your organization's strengths and weaknesses helps you evaluate your shelter, capitalize on what is working, and address what needs to be improved. This insight is integral to effective strategic planning for your organization and for specific programs. You will also be able to tout your best points to funders and note how you will manage shortcomings. For example, perhaps your operations are running smoothly and you have strong community backing, but your organization lacks financial management skills. You might have a strong case for seeking support from a foundation that offers capacity development grants for training. If you can show how better technology would enhance your popular behavior training program and provide visibility for a corporate sponsor, a local business might donate equipment or volunteer support.

Assessing your organization's strengths and weaknesses is an ongoing process, not a one-time project. As your external environment shifts, you will have to find new ways to respond to emerging needs in the community or changes in other organizations' strategies. And as your own organization grows and evolves, its strengths and weaknesses will change, too.

How can your organization use the information it collects to determine its strengths and weaknesses? Answering these questions can help you make the connection:

- How does your community perceive your organization and its programs? How successful have you been in attracting the population as clients and donors?

- How well do your programs and services meet community needs? Are you reaching different neighborhoods and demographic groups effectively?

- How do you compare to similar organizations locally and nationally? Where do you see relative strengths in your organization that your community and potential funders would value? (To evaluate these organizations, read their materials, explore their web sites, visit their offices, and read local news coverage of them.)

- Do you have the right personnel, skills, culture, technology, facilities, and funding to meet current and emerging needs?

Press for meaningful answers. Do not just say, "We have good people." Be specific. Are your staff and volunteers client-service-oriented, knowledgeable in resolving animal behavior problems, or well connected in the community? Why are these qualities important to your community and to your organization? Often it can be difficult for the staff and directors to assess strengths and weaknesses thoroughly and objectively. Some teams are too positive, accentuating all the good news and ignoring the problems. Other groups are extremely self-critical, dwelling on everything they do wrong and giving little credit for what they have to offer.

To create a realistic assessment of strengths and weaknesses, follow these tips:

- Identify and consider three to five of your organization's biggest successes in the past few years. What strengths contributed to these victories? Look at your disappointments to discover weaknesses.

- Involve selected members of your community in your "strengths and weaknesses" evaluation. Include representatives of key constituencies who bring diverse perspectives to your discussion.

Asking for Opinions

One of the most helpful ways to get an accurate picture of your strengths and weaknesses is to ask people outside your organization. "Primary research" is research you undertake to generate original data rather than existing data gathered by others. Interviews, focus groups, and surveys not only can validate your organization's strengths and weaknesses, but they can also provide critical, community-specific information that you cannot find in "pre-packaged" reports. You can use this information to improve your decision making, define your plans, and justify funding.

- If you want to set priorities for your organization and demonstrate the need to increase resources, you could ask community leaders what they view as the most pressing animal issues and survey the public to rank the results in order of priority.

- If you want to define high-impact campaigns and show why you believe they will succeed, you could interview people about why they have not taken a particular action (e.g., adoption, spay/neuter, animal licensing) and what it would take for them to do so.

- If you want to develop effective outreach programs and justify financial assistance, you could meet with representatives of different neighborhoods or demographic groups to learn how they perceive your organization.

■ If you want to determine what other animal care organizations have achieved with spay/neuter clinics so you can persuade the public and government of your community's need for one, you could ask executive directors of animal care organizations in communities like yours to share their experiences.

■ If you want to assess the value of staff training in client service to consider additional investment, you could survey visitors to your animal care organization to learn what proportion of them are satisfied with their experience (before and after training).

■ If you want to create more effective fund-raising campaigns, you could talk to donors about why they support your shelter and to non-donors about what might motivate them to contribute.

■ If you want to test whether your publications create the desired impression so you can identify potential enhancements and seek support for implementation, you could gather a group of people from the target audience to review the materials, discuss their reaction, and suggest improvements.

Here are questions that one animal care organization asked community residents to help the organization prioritize programs:

■ What services and products should be available at our shelter?

■ What should be the animal shelter's top three goals?

■ What should "excellent client service" mean for our animal shelter?

Making Room for Market Research

Before you dismiss market research as an expensive option, consider how much it costs your organization in time, dollars, and morale to pursue efforts that *don't* work. Think about where you may miss out on funding opportunities because you cannot demonstrate needs or your organization's impact clearly. Investing in good market research can be one of the best uses of your scarce resources.

Affordable assistance does exist. Consider these sources:

■ members of your organization who may be market research professionals

■ local market research firms with reduced-fee or pro bono services for nonprofits

- marketing students or professors at local
  universities, preferably at the graduate level

- the Humane Research Council (*www.humaneresearch.org*),
  a nonprofit market research service provider that
  specializes in animal-protection issues

Ask the following questions as you develop a simple market research plan to help your organization get and stay on track:

What Information Do You Need?

Don't ask questions unless you know how you will use the results. Double-check that you are collecting data that will help you document the need for services, support the benefit of proposed solutions, and choose the best options or measure outcomes.

Who Is the Target Audience?

Often you will need to hear from representatives of your entire community. In other situations, you might focus on government, animal care professionals, parents, educators, or a selected demographic group.

What Type of Results Do You Want?

Qualitative research involves posing unstructured, exploratory questions to small numbers of people to deepen understanding of a problem. Interviewing community leaders and meeting with small groups of citizens or members of a target audience are methods you can use for qualitative research. These efforts reveal surface impressions and ideas, but they do not enable you to draw quantified conclusions (e.g., "X percent believe").

Quantitative research involves collecting large samples of objective data—such as when surveying the public to rank priorities and asking visitors to rate customer satisfaction. Your survey needs to include at least thirty and preferably one hundred to two hundred respondents for each group you want to analyze separately, such as men vs. women.

How Will You Collect Data?

- Interviews involve questioning a small number of people
  verbally. This can be an easy way to get input, but you
  must word questions and choose individuals carefully.

- Focus groups are informal discussions with eight
  to twelve participants, led by a skilled moderator
  who guides but does not influence the interaction.

- Surveys gather input from many individuals, using
  questionnaires delivered by mail, in person, by
  telephone, or online.

—*Caryn Ginsberg*

Strategic Planning Basics

Astrategic plan provides direction and steps, clarifies organizational values, examines environmental factors, involves constituents, sets measurable goals and strategies, and defines program and support activities for the organization as a whole. This communications document serves as a referral source and "user's manual" for staff, board members, and committees. Think of it as the road map for your organization's journey.

An effective strategic plan creates awareness of resources necessary to design, implement, monitor, and evaluate your organization's programs and strategies, thereby strengthening accountability and ensuring that your organization meets a community need. Having a plan and working the plan ensures the most effective usc of financial and human resources and keeps everyone focused on the mission and destination to maximize your success.

Your animal care organization's strategic plan should accomplish the following:

- develop/review organization's mission

- chart the direction and steps

- examine the environment

- set measurable goals and strategies

- define the program and agency support activities

- define the organization's niche in the community

- outline responsibilities and timelines

- estimate resources needed and resource availability

- define indicators for success

Your organization's plan, like most strategic plans, should encompass three to five years of planning and be evaluated annually.

Pulling in the Right People

Developing a strategic plan is never a one-person job. A successful plan requires the participation and "buy-in" of many key players in your organization. Make sure you involve your organization's board members, executive director, development officer, critical management staff, and key constituents in the process.

In small to mid-size organizations, this group can develop the strategic plan at a retreat. Larger organizations typically establish a formal committee to develop the plan. But before any planning group can start strategizing, participants must first identify and agree on the organization's values—the beliefs and principles that describe how your organization functions and makes decisions. This set of values will guide decision making and performance.

As with any major initiative, the strategic planning process will be smoother and more effective if it is managed by an outside facilitator. Consider a professional planner, outside consultant, or even a volunteer with proven leadership and organization skills. Check with your local volunteer center or other nonprofit groups for referrals.

Assigning Homework

Before gathering group members around a table, send a questionnaire to participants to assess the environment. This situational analysis examines your organization's strengths and weaknesses and external opportunities and threats. Internal strengths and weaknesses refer to available resources (staff, facilities, equipment, etc.; volunteer leadership; financial and human resources; and customer service). External analysis examines your organization's role in the community (changing community needs, social and economic factors as well as technological, philanthropic, and political trends that can affect your programs). Set a deadline for questionnaires to be returned to the facilitator for compilation before the big meeting or retreat. Compiling the results on a flip chart, with an overhead projector, or into a PowerPoint presentation will start the process.

Sample Board Member Questionnaire

1. Our mission statement is:

2. Our mission statement is acceptable (Yes or No), or it should be changed to reflect the following:

3. Our greatest strengths are:

4. Our major weakness is:

5. What is happening in our community that will affect our organization in a positive way?

6. What is happening in our community that will affect our organization in a negative way?

7. What perception does the community have of our organization?

8. Is there something you think we should do to improve the image of our organization in the community?

9. Why do you serve on the board?

10. To reach our full potential as an organization I should:

11. What are the top three goals our organization should focus on?

12. Where would you like to see our organization in the next ten years?

13. What strengths do you bring to the organization: wealth, wisdom, or work?

14. What are your expectations for this retreat?

Molding Your Mission Statement

Using the results of your environmental assessment, begin the strategic planning retreat by reviewing (or, if necessary, developing) the organization's mission statement—the introductory statement of accountability. Your organization's mission statement should apprise the audience of the organization's direction and indicate that it knows where it is going. The mission tells the purpose (why the organization exists and what it does); the method (how the organization fulfills its purpose); and the values (the principles or beliefs that guide the organization as it pursues its purpose). Here are a few examples to help your organization create or evaluate its own statement:

- "The mission of The Humane Society of the United States is to create a humane and sustainable world for all animals, including people, through education, advocacy, and the promotion of respect and compassion."

- "Guided by the humane ethic, it is the mission of The Marin Humane Society to protect animals from neglect, abuse, and exploitation, to advocate for their interests and welfare, and to inspire awareness and compassion for all living things."

- "The mission of the Houston SPCA is to promote respect for all animals and free them from suffering and abuse."

- "The mission of the Michigan Humane Society is to provide the highest quality service and compassion to the animals entrusted to our care, to measurably reduce companion animal overpopulation, and to take a leadership role in promoting humane values for the benefit of all animals."

The assessment may reveal a need to revise or update your mission statement. Be sure to evaluate whether the statement is still relevant, taking into consideration trends and issues currently facing your organization and community. If not, explore what changes need to be made.

Going for the Goal

Using your mission statement as a guide, focus next on those issues your organization wants to address now and in the years ahead. Have your board base its decisions about the organization's goals on information researched and prepared by staff (or those assigned to this task).

Make sure the selected goals are realistic and achievable. You want to be successful—too many goals, or goals you cannot accomplish realistically within the projected time frame, can end in failure. You will build more excitement and momentum if you can accomplish your goals and return to the drawing board to set new ones. Success breeds success.

After establishing specific goals, match them with programs and activities. Then identify key tasks and required resources, both human and financial, needed to carry out those plans. (Typically staff will prepare a timetable for these programs and activities for planning participants to review. But if you have time at the planning meeting or retreat, try establishing some general timelines and assignments for your action plan.)

Living Within Your Means

A passionate group committed to helping animals is a wonderful thing, but it is common for such groups to plan lofty programs without first ensuring they have the resources needed to carry them out. To make sure that your organization lives within its means, analyze income, estimate resource requirements, and develop budget projections. With this information in hand, you can review your strategic plan for feasibility more accurately. Because of available financial and human resources, you may need to adjust timetables and programs to ensure that you have a workable plan.

Wrapping It Up

Assign an individual or committee to assemble all of the information from your strategic planning retreat into draft form to present to the board of directors. Because board and staff worked together, making decisions throughout the process, the actual plan is a detailed articulation of determined consensus. The board should be ready now to adopt the plan as a policy document for the organization. Once the plan is adopted as policy, you have a road map to plan the rest of the trip.

The road map will help your animal care organization achieve its goals only if you use it. Staff members usually manage implementation with regular progress reports to the board. (In small, grassroots organizations without paid staff, the board and volunteers will manage the plan.) If problems arise as the plan is carried out, the organization can make necessary adjustments.

The strategic plan is critical to development of specific annual work plans, and staff and volunteers implement activities in accordance with the plan. One of the final steps in the strategic plan is completing a budget and setting fund-raising goals. With the strategic plan, implementation, and monitoring in place, you are now ready to create the detailed annual development plan.

—Karen Medicus

Board Development Basics

Board recruitment and selection is an ongoing process based on identifying needs and recognizing and recruiting the right people to fill those needs. To fill a board vacancy, many organizations select a friend of one of the current members or someone who volunteers at the organization. But not everyone who works with your organization belongs on the board. For example, it is difficult for a person take off his "volunteer hat" and replace it with the "governance hat" when the individual favors certain programs and employees. Such a situation can also confuse other volunteers and staff, who may expect the new board member to side with them. The result can be hurt feelings or, worse, a board whose governance becomes severely undermined.

Identifying skill sets needed to build a strong board of directors and finding the right people to serve is the only way to build a stable, productive, and emotionally balanced board. As *Star Trek*'s Mr. Spock said, "The needs of the many outweigh the needs of the few—or the one." Staying focused on the health of the organization as a whole and the mission of saving animals far outweighs the needs of one or a few counterproductive board members. A successful business, whether for-profit or nonprofit, is built on the skills those involved bring to the organization. Identify the desired characteristics needed to make your organization successful (see chapter 5).

Telling It Like It Is

Be honest when recruiting new board members. Do not tell them that serving on the board will not take much time or that they do not have to do fund-raising. Be up front about the amount of time involved and the financial commitment required.

To help current and prospective board members better understand their roles and responsibilities, provide detailed job descriptions for all board positions. Be sure to answer these basic issues:

- What are board members' duties?

- What is expected of board members?

- What skills are needed?

- Does the organization offer training?

- What time of day or night is most of the work done?

- With whom will board members interact?

Many board members lose interest because they were given unrealistic goals, poorly detailed responsibilities, and insufficient feedback and recognition.

Formalizing the Selection Process

Typically, board volunteers are recruited through a formal process with specific policies and procedures and elected by board vote.

The nominating committee is one of the most important committees in the organization. This committee is responsible for developing board and committee chair job descriptions, the board manual, recruitment, board applications, screening, presentation to the board, orientation, and performance evaluation. The nominating committee should be busy all year long—not just before the annual election.

Design the selection process to fit your organization's needs and follow it for every nomination. The selection process for new board members can include:

1. completion of application form

2. contact with two references provided by the applicant

3. personal interview with the nominating committee

4. facility tour

Questionnaires and Sample Board Positions

After designing the process, develop the questionnaire. Sample fill-in-the-blank requests can include:

1. Who is your employer?

2. What is your spouse or partner's profession?

3. Describe your education, including any degrees earned.

4. Detail your pet history (list any pets owned in the last ten years and include any pets that may be contained [fish, gerbil, rabbit, etc.]).

5. Are your pets spayed or neutered?

6. What is/was the name of the veterinarian?

7. Have you been an officer, board member, or volunteer of an animal welfare or animal rights group?

8. Are you currently a member of this/these organization(s)? If not, why did you leave?

9. Why do you want to be a member of the board of directors of the XYZ Humane Society?

10. What talents, skills, abilities, etc., could you contribute to the board of directors and the organization?

11. The XYZ Humane Society meets on the second
    Wednesday of each month from noon to 1:30 p.m.
    Can you attend these monthly meetings regularly?
    Please discuss your availability (time and effort)
    beyond these monthly meetings.

12. What improvements or changes would you like
    to see occur at the XYZ Humane Society?

13. What concerns or questions do you have
    on the topic of euthanasia?

14. In your opinion, what is the role of a board member?

15. Have you served on other boards? If so, please list them.

The nominating committee should also develop a list of questions to ask during the interview. These can include:

1. What do you feel we, as a society, can do
   to prevent animal cruelty and suffering?

2. If you were a board member of the XYZ Humane
   Society, how would you respond if another board
   member disagreed with you on a particular issue?

3. Please share some of your ideas about
   fund-raising activities for our organization.

The nominating committee also must be prepared to provide detailed information on member positions and responsibilities, such as maintaining knowledge of the organization and personal commitment to its goals and objectives. Sample job descriptions for board positions are available at *www.boardsource.org* (search on "job description").

The nominating committee is responsible not just for selecting competent board members, but also for evaluating their performance on the board. Here are some sample criteria the nominating committee could include in board member evaluation ratings:

- demonstrates ability to work cooperatively and respectfully
  as a team member of the board (not just as an individual)

- demonstrates regular and punctual attendance
  at board meetings

- supports the organization's special events throughout the
  year as a donor, working volunteer, and/or participant

- demonstrates support of the organization's philosophy by
  exhibiting responsible companion animal guardianship
  with animals in his or her care

- demonstrates understanding of the strategic plan and
  actively participates in efforts to accomplish plan goals

- demonstrates a clear understanding of the vision
  and mission of the organization

- participates in meaningful, respectful discussions at board meetings

- actively participates on at least one committee

- refrains from developing close, personal relationships with the staff and does not interfere with day-to-day details of staff work

- accepts responsibilities and duties as requested by the president/chair

- meets the required financial commitment in a timely manner

Helping New Members Get Adjusted

After your organization has successfully recruited new board members, you need to ensure their success by providing orientation and training. A typical orientation—usually conducted by the board president/chair and the executive director (or sometimes by the executive director and development director)—includes:

1. Distributing a three-ring binder containing biographies of the current board members and their terms; last audited financial report; most current profit and loss statement; current year budget; financial and investment policies (and other relevant financial reports); copies of minutes (last six months) with associated reports; board job descriptions; employee manual; board manual (if you have one); bylaws; articles of incorporation; IRS determination letter; mission and vision statement; strategic plan; policy on conflicts of interest; insurance policy coverage; Form 990; current major donor list; staff listing; web site information; annual meeting schedule; organizational history; brief biography of the executive director; organization chart; current standard operating procedures (for day-to-day operations); latest press clippings about the organization; and stationery, brochures, and promotional materials (which can be placed in the pockets of the notebook).

2. Reviewing the contents of the binder with the new board member and encouraging discussion and questions.

3. Briefing the new board member on current issues facing the organization and items coming up for board vote.

4. Conducting a tour of the facility and giving a brief overview of operating procedures. Consider having board members participate in ride-alongs and shadow key staff to observe the organization's daily reality.

5. Introducing the new board member to the staff.

6. Showing a short video on board responsibilities
   (available through Board Source: *www.boardsource.org*)
   or on one of your organization's programs.

Another way you can help your new members feel more comfortable and adapt more quickly is through a buddy system: assign a current, experienced board member to work with a new member.

Meeting Members' Meeting Needs

To attract and keep dynamic, professional board members, your organization must hold productive monthly board meetings that last no more than an hour and a half (longer times can be productive if you are only meeting quarterly). Board meetings that drag on with committee work for hours will discourage those movers and shakers you want on your board.

Board meetings are for decision making through voting, not for committee work. Committees should meet separately to look at issues, programs, and events in-depth and report their findings to the board with a recommendation for action. If the board wants more information or feels action should not be taken yet, it then gives direction to the committee on the additional information it wants. The committee meets again to prepare another presentation for the board at the next regular meeting.

Running a short, successful meeting does not require board members to keep quiet and rubber-stamp all decisions. In fact, many board decisions are not made unanimously. Board members contribute varying and, at times, controversial perspectives to deliberations. These new and different ideas assist the board in reaching an objective and balanced decision. During the voting process, if a board member strongly disagrees with a motion and votes against it or abstains from voting, that vote should be recorded in the meeting minutes.

Board decisions are based on majority rule, which automatically creates compromises and, occasionally, dissenting opinions. Make sure that your board members understand that once a decision is made, the board speaks with one voice, and individual board members are obligated to present this view to the outside world.

Getting Everyone to Get Along

Although tough questions and differing opinions should not be stifled, rudeness, aggressiveness, and hostile behavior have no place in the boardroom. The board must work as a team, and each member of the team must contribute to creating a positive atmosphere for deliberation and decision making. According to BoardSource, to keep the board running smoothly, the president/chair of the board should:

■ Ensure that all opinions on issues are welcome.

■ Immediately stop negative personal comments or insinuations and direct the discussion back to issues.

■ Have a private discussion with the disruptive board member to find out the reasons for the behavior and to explain the detrimental effects of this behavior.

■ Give the disgruntled board member meaningful
assignments and expect results.

If unacceptable behavior continues, consider making the situation a full board issue
and discuss removal if the member declines to resign voluntarily.

Making Room for Change

Every nonprofit board experiences a life cycle. When an organization is newly formed and operating
at the grassroots level, the board of directors does everything—the day-to-day work, fund-raising,
and governance. Typically, this group comprises dedicated, compassionate, and focused individuals
who see a need in their community and set out to address it. When their hard work and dedication
pay off and the organization grows successfully, the board members realize that they can no longer
do everything, and it becomes necessary to hire staff. This can be a painful process, especially for
the founder or founding members, as board members struggle to let go of the day-to-day work and
focus on the next steps: building a governance and development board, setting policy, raising
money, and allowing the professional paid staff to handle operations. Some organizations never
make it past this step and stay in an endless cycle of hiring and firing staff. When an organization
does make it past this step, it can celebrate its success in building a strong governance board that
will guide the organization into the future. The saying, the "only thing that is constant in life is
change," is true for boards, too. Flexibility is the key to successful growth.

—Karen Medicus

Appendix D

Sample Forms

Appendix D.1

Sample Development Plan Giving Trends Evaluation

	2000		2001		2002		2003	
	Number of Gifts	Dollars	Number of Gifts	Dollars	Number of Gifts	Dollars	Number of Gifts	Dollars
$5,000 and above	14	$331,151	13	$145,248	11	$110,612	17	$216,480
$2,500–$4,999	5	$14,969	8	$23,427	8	$23,533	10	$28,700
$1,000–$2,499	48	$56,810	66	$84,443	91	$112,179	103	$127,417
$500–$999	66	$36,694	91	$52,997	111	$64,035	124	$74,523
$250–$499	84	$25,047	122	$38,280	155	$49,335	147	$47,822
$100–$249	563	$69,805	639	$82,565	857	$111,243	1,004	$129,842
$50–$99	993	$55,928	921	$53,668	1,314	$73,448	1,561	$83,975
$25–$49	1,988	$58,697	2,069	$59,932	3,275	$91,929	3,879	$104,450
$1–$24	3,254	$42,528	3,049	$38,630	4,401	$55,045	4,832	$59,917
	7,015	$691,629	6,978	$579,190	10,223	$691,359	11,677	$873,126

Courtesy Maryland SPCA

Appendix D.1 Sample Development Plan Giving Trends Evaluation

Appendix D.2

Sample Development Plan Giving History Evaluation

Source	Actual 2000	Actual 2001	Change 00–01	Actual 2002	Change 01–02	Actual 2003	Change 02–03	Change 2000–2003
Auto Donations	$64,525	$81,785	27%	$41,115	-50%	$32,620	-21%	-49%
Bequests	$230,014	$38,477	-83%	$17,000	-56%	$34,382	102%	-85%
Board Giving	$37,000	$45,000	22%	$49,036	9%	$48,485	-1%	31%
Cages	$8,250	$9,751	18%	$5,000	-49%	$4,645	-7%	-44%
Calendar	$ -	$ -		$59,360		$69,875	18%	
Corporations & Foundations	$71,000	$32,105	-55%	$38,957	21%	$111,521	186%	57%
Direct Mail	$16,997	$74,860	340%	$160,628	115%	$191,973	20%	1029%
Electronic Fund	$80	$1,649	1961%	$2,456	49%	$3,275	33%	3993%
Honor/Memorial	$13,798	$20,850	51%	$16,911	-19%	$36,550	116%	165%
Howl-o-Ween Hop	$47,683	$59,927	26%	$60,000	0%	$63,000	5%	32%
Major Donor Appeal	$40,647	$26,270	-35%	$26,216	0%	$47,544	81%	17%
Newsletter	$15,013	$15,901	6%	$17,288	9%	$22,711	31%	51%
Past Board/ Volunteers	$1,500	$3,533	136%	$9,155	159%	$9,170	0%	511%
Walkathon	$115,000	$154,000	34%	$157,000	2%	$139,000	-11%	21%
Workplace Giving	$10,877	$30,989	185%	$28,738	-7%	$33,054	15%	204%
Unsolicited/ Other	$30,913	$75,414	144%	$74,861	-1%	$91,015	22%	194%
Total	$703,297	$670,511	-5%	$763,720	14%	$938,819	23%	33%
Total, excluding bequests	$473,283	$632,034	34%	$746,720	18%	$904,437	21%	91%

Courtesy Maryland SPCA

Fund-Raising for Animal Care Organizations

Appendix D.3

Sample Development Plan Evaluation Process

Priority	Activity	Date	Time Frame	Staff Resources	Volunteer Resources	Gross Revenue	Net Revenue
	March for the Animals	Last Sunday in March	Planning Aug–Mar; data entry Mar–June	Director of Volunteers & Events, Development Coordinator, Program Coordinator	Committee of 8–10, 2–3 volunteers do data entry; 30 volunteers day of event	$190,000	$168,000
	Pet Calendar	Published in September	Planning Jan–June; kickoff event in Sept., sales until 12/31	Director of Development, Ass't. Dir. of Development	Committee of 8–10 volunteers	$70,000	$39,000
	Howl-o-Ween Hop	Last Saturday in October	Planning April–Oct.	Ass't. Dir. of Development, Dir. of Development	Committee of 8–10 volunteers; 15 addi'tl volunteers weekend of event	$63,000	$42,000
	Direct Mail	8x/year	Ongoing	Director of Development, Ass't. Dir. of Development	None	$180,000	$100,000
	Major Donors	Fall	Oct.–early Dec.	Director of Development, Executive Director	Development Committee	$30,000	$1,000
	Planned Giving	Ongoing	Ongoing	Director of Development	None	$20,000	$19,000
					TOTAL	$553,000	$369,000

Courtesy Maryland SPCA

Appendix D.4

Sample Development Plan Gift Projections

Source	Projected 2004	Actual 2004	Projected 2005	Projected 2006	Projected 2007
Auto Donations	$50,000	$50,028	$30,000	$15,000	$ -
Bequests	$20,000	$98,485	$20,000	$20,000	$25,000
Board Giving	$46,000	$57,094	$50,000	$50,000	$50,000
Cages	$2,000	$2,000	$1,500	$1,500	$1,500
Calendar	$68,000	$82,920	$80,000	$72,000	$74,000
Corporations & Foundations	$35,000	$86,469	$50,000	$50,000	$50,000
Direct Mail	$180,000	$187,441	$210,000	$215,000	$220,000
Electronic Fund	$3,000	$3,852	$3,200	$3,400	$3,400
Honor/Memorial	$22,000	$30,988	$25,000	$25,000	$25,000
Howl-o-Ween Hop	$65,000	$61,200	$68,000	$70,000	$70,000
Major Donor Appeal	$40,000	$27,249	$50,000	$65,000	$75,000
Newsletter	$17,000	$20,383	$18,000	$18,000	$18,000
Past Board/ Volunteers	$9,500	$10,935	$10,000	$10,000	$10,000
Walk-a-thon	$180,000	$197,569	$195,000	$203,000	$214,000
Workplace Giving	$38,000	$39,990	$40,000	$42,000	$45,000
Unsolicited/Other	$55,000	$131,660	$55,000	$55,000	$55,000
Total	**$830,500**	**$1,088,263**	**$905,700**	**$914,900**	**$935,900**
Total, excluding bequests	**$810,500**	**$989,778**	**$885,700**	**$894,900**	**$910,900**

Courtesy Maryland SPCA

Appendix D.5

Sample Conflict-of-Interest Policy

Los Angeles County Animal Care Foundation Policy 002: Conflict of Interest

Whereas, board members have a fiduciary responsibility to the Foundation to act in the best interest of the Foundation, and board members must administer the Foundation's affairs fairly and impartially without opportunity for personal gain;

Resolved, the following Conflict-of-Interest policy for the board members of the Los Angeles County Animal Care Foundation shall be enacted and subsequently enforced until amended or repealed:

No board member of the Los Angeles County Animal Care Foundation (Foundation) shall derive any personal profit or gain, directly or indirectly, by reason of his or her participation with the Foundation. Each individual shall disclose to the Foundation any personal interest that he or she may have in any matter pending before the Foundation and he/she shall not participate in the vote affecting that decision, and the decision must be made and/or ratified by the full board. Such transactions include, but are not limited to:

- An ownership interest in a vendor from whom the Foundation buys goods and services
- An interest in property the Foundation is buying or leasing
- Doing business with a board member's family member, close friend, or business partner
- Holding management positions, serving on the board of or being formally employed by any third party dealing with the Foundation
- Receiving compensation for services for individual transactions involving the Foundation
- Using Foundation resources—including personnel, equipment and supplies—for other than Foundation-sponsored activities, programs and purposes
- Receiving anything that could be considered a gift from any third party dealing with the Foundation

Any board member of the Foundation who is an officer, board member, a committee member or staff member of a borrower organization or a loan applicant agency shall identify his or her affiliation with such agency or agencies; further, in connection with any credit policy committee or board action specifically directed to that agency, he/she shall not participate in the decision affecting that agency and the decision must be made and/or ratified by the full board.

Any board member of the Foundation shall refrain from obtaining any list of Foundation donors for personal or private solicitation purposes at any time during the term of their affiliation.

Relationships with related parties will be considered only under the same terms and selection processes as with any other vendor or entity.

Enacted: February 2003

I acknowledge and agree to follow this Conflict-of-Interest policy

_____   _____

Board Member   Date

Appendix D.6

Sample Job Description for Director of Development

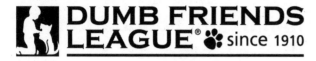

DUMB FRIENDS LEAGUE® 🐾 since 1910

Title: **Director of Development/Community Relations**

Department: **Development/Community Relations**

Purpose of Position: Directs the design and implementation of all fund-raising and community relations activities for the League, to include strategic planning and departmental budget preparation. Provides quality people care in accordance with the League's mission, goals, and management philosophy.

This position reports to: President

This position directly supervises: Annual Gifts Manager, Special Events Coordinator, Capital Campaign Administrators, Development Assistant

Accountability/Project: **Measures of Accomplishments**

1. Fund-Raising Management
      A. Total Net Revenue Raised
      B. # of New Funding Sources
      C. # of Projects Managed
      D. Relationship with Board and Committees

Raises operating revenue for the League, including new and established campaigns. Activities include prospecting, researching, communication with League departments and staff, and appropriate committees and Board. Prospects include renewal donors, corporations, foundations, and individuals. Responsibilities also include proposal writing, cultivation of major donors, and planned giving, to include foundations, corporations, and individuals.

2. Donor Cultivation and Marketing
      A. Timeliness
      B. Quality
      C. # of New Projects/Ideas Cultivated
      D. # of Qualified Prospects

Directs and manages the Board's/Development Committee's role in major donor cultivation. Develops and maintains relationships with donors, to include foundations, corporations, community organizations and individuals. Provides an annual comprehensive analysis of department and fund-raising programs. Provides analysis and evaluation for individual programs on an as-needed basis. Plans and directs the marketing of fund-raising efforts to Board, staff, and community. Plans and initiates new ideas, innovative and creative solutions, and new projects.

Accountability/Project:	Measures of Accomplishments
3. **Publicity and Publications**	A. **# of Media Contacts** B. **Quality** C. **Timeliness** D. **Effectiveness**

Promotes public awareness of the League's mission, position, goals, and services. Oversees staff responsible for the professional design, editing, and production of all League printed materials. Works with advertising agencies and various vendors to create print, radio, TV, and other advertising to advance awareness of the League. Plans and oversees outreach efforts, which combine and capitalize on the various programs within the department.

4. **Program Management**	A. **Quality** B. **Program Growth** C. **Feedback**

Oversees the Humane Education and Pets Are Welcome programs to ensure quality/content of programming delivered to improve public understanding and awareness of League and animal welfare issues as well as facilitate pet-friendly housing for Denver-area residents. Develops ideas and works with staff to enhance program growth and administration.

5. **Staff/Volunteer Management**	A. **Accountabilities of Supervised Staff Met** B. **Appropriateness of Coaching, Review, and Training of Staff** C. **Development Plans in Place and Being Met** D. **Timely Reviews** E. **Feedback**

Directs and supervises development and community relations staff and volunteers in the performance of their respective responsibilities within the department. Coaches staff by providing regular, ongoing feedback and timely performance evaluations. Assures staff is trained and coached to a level necessary to achieve League's mission, goals, and management philosophy. Monitors safety compliance of staff and takes immediate action to correct hazards. Develops annual goals for department staff that include timelines, procedures, and accountabilities to be accomplished in meeting future plans and goals. Provides guidance, direction, and resolutions for problems or staff issues. Recommends training programs for staff to ensure development and continuous improvement in the performance of their duties. Maintains a professional fund-raising and community relations staff by providing training and motivation in a team climate. Approves departmental vacation/leave requests.

6. **Budget Management**	A. **Under/Over Budget** B. **Timeliness** C. **Accuracy** D. **Feedback**

continued...

Effectively manages resources, both people and dollars, for the maximum benefit to the departments and the League. Prepares and executes departmental budget annually, to include projected income and expenses. Prepares and submits annual income and expenditure budget for the department to president for review, recommendations, and approval. Administers and monitors revenues and expenses in relation to annual budget. Compiles summary reports for Board presentations. Discusses budget projections and accounting procedures with direct reports to resolve any discrepancies.

Accountability/Project:	Measures of Accomplishments
7. Special Projects	A. Quality B. Feedback C. # of Accomplishments D. Timeliness

Serves on special committees at the request of the Board, president, etc., projects or teams. Special projects may or may not be limited to projects related to development and could include special training projects and events such as all-staff meetings.

8. People Care	A. Feedback B. Responsiveness C. Cooperation D. Problem Solving

Ensures quality people care is provided to patrons, visitors, staff, and volunteers at the League. Assists staff in situations requiring immediate problem solving. Takes control of situations that could be potentially damaging to the professional image of the League. Recommends continuous improvements in the adoption and pet supply areas related to services provided.

9. Additional Management Expectations

Communications
Is visible to staff, communicates with director on significant developments within the department. Attends necessary meetings. Communicates pertinent information to staff, manager, and director and ensures that supervisors communicate effectively with line staff. Communicates and problem solves with other managers.

Organizational Development
Ensures that policies and procedures are followed. Develops new ideas with staff. Develops and follows timelines for annual plans and projects and is accountable for staff's decisions and actions. Supports management and discusses differences privately.

Development
Encourages use of volunteers, solicitation of monetary, and use of in-kind, donations whenever possible.

Fiscal Responsibility
Maintains control of budgets, including approving invoices and preparing financial and/or statistical reports as needed.

Staff Management

Uses performance-based management when counseling and evaluating staff and sets measurable goals for employee growth. Submits evaluations on time and encourages continuing education for staff as it relates to the organization's needs. Recognizes good performance and counsels staff to correct problems.

Availability

Is flexible with scheduling and is available when away from the facility as needed to meet the needs of the organization.

Position Specifications: (Education, Experience, Certification, and Knowledge/Skills/Abilities)

Required: Bachelor's degree in nonprofit management or related field such as communications, public relations, marketing, or business and minimum of five years of proven successful experience in fund-raising and development. Excellent verbal and written skills are mandatory, as are organizational skills, attention to detail, and ability to be self-motivated and disciplined. One year of supervisory experience. Ability to work with wide diversity of individuals, including high-level corporate executives and managers. Computer-literate in a Windows environment.

Desired: Prior successful experience managing and securing major and planned gifts in a nonprofit environment. Experience working with volunteers.

Work Conditions:

May work in an area with a high noise level. Potentially subject to animal bites and scratches. Occasional lifting up to seventy-five pounds with reasonable accommodations. Also performs work in an office setting. Frequent walking, standing, bending, and stooping. **Expected to work extended hours as needed.** May be required to maintain availability when away from the shelter as directed by department director or president.

This position description in no way states or implies that these are the only duties to be performed by the employee occupying this position. Employees will be required to perform any other job-related duties required by their supervisor. This document does not create an employment contract implied or otherwise, other than an at-will relationship.

Approved:

_____   _____
Human Resources Manager   Date

_____   _____
President   Date

Reviewed:

_____   _____
Position's Incumbent   Date

Revised: 4/1/03

Appendix D.7

Selecting Development Software

Going over these questions can help you select the development software system that meets your organization's needs.

For "prospects and donors" tracking:

1. Can you track prospects and donors in the same manner for easy conversion?
2. Can you track individual and organizational prospects and donors?
3. Can you track the personal information you need about a prospect/donor?
4. Can you track and make use of multiple addresses and telephone numbers for donors/prospects?
5. Can you track the rating information you need about a prospect/donor?
6. Can you track the prospect/donor's relationship to your organization?
7. Can you track as many prospect/donor relationships with other organizations as you want?
8. Can you track as many prospect/donor activities, skills, and/or interests as you want?
9. Can you track prospect/donor memberships?
10. Can you produce customized donor master lists?
11. Can you recognize certain donors?
12. Can you analyze donors based on a time frame you define?

For "donations" tracking and record-keeping:

1. Can you track as many gifts and/or pledges as you want for each donor?
2. Can you maintain gift and/or pledge history for as long as you want?
3. Can you track the campaign to which a gift and/or pledge applies?
4. Can you track gift and/or pledge and date received?
5. Can you track whether a gift and/or pledge is restricted or unrestricted?
6. Can you track the method through which you acquired gift and/or pledge?
7. Can you track the solicitor through whom you acquired the gift and/or pledge?
8. Can you track organizations that match gifts and/or pledges?
9. Can you set up monthly, quarterly, semiannual, annual, biannual, or irregular pledge payment cycles?
10. Can you track data on when pledge payments are expected or were received?
11. Can you track balance due on pledges?
12. Can you track total of all gifts?
13. Can you check gift/pledge entries for accuracy before posting to permanent history?
14. Can you produce gift/pledge transmittal reports?
15. Can you produce timely, personalized pledge cards and reminders?
16. Can you track past-due pledges?

17. Can you track paid pledges?

18. Can you analyze campaign income—current, predicted, and/or forecast—within the time frames you define?

19. Can you produce gift/pledge range reports?

For "campaign and solicitors" tracking and record-keeping:

1. Can you track multiple campaigns simultaneously?

2. Can you organize and track the awareness process?

3. Can you assign solicitors to campaigns?

4. Can you organize solicitors into teams?

5. Can you assign prospects/donors to solicitors?

6. Can you track solicitor spheres of influence?

7. Can you produce timely solicitor tools?

8. Can you thank your solicitors?

9. Can you track solicitor productivity?

For "mailings and other contacts" tracking and record-keeping:

1. Can you target personalized solicitations based on criteria you select?

2. Can you take advantage of bulk-mail rates?

3. Can you track contact with prospects/donors?

4. Can you track mailing types?

5. Can you maintain a tickler system for future contact?

For "custom reports" tracking:

1. Can you produce reports based on criteria you select?

2. Can you make "and" selections? (e.g., list all donors who live in an area and gave $100)

3. Can you make "or" selections? (e.g., list all donors who live in an area or gave $100)

4. Can you use any information you track as selection criteria?

5. Can you make as many selection passes as you want?

6. Can you sort results in the order you want?

For "miscellaneous" procedures:

1. Can you change field names or lengths?

2. Can you define your own fields?

3. Can you add or skip fields?

4. Can you define your own codes?

5. Can you verify online (on screen during entry) that your code is accurate?

6. Can you look up your codes online (on screen during entry)?

7. Can you import information from and/or export information to other automated systems?

continued…

For "general" uses:

1. How long does it take to enter, process, and print information?

2. Is the software easy to use? What does it cost?

3. Does the software have full word-processing capability?

4. Do you need to learn to operate database management software before you can make full use of the development management software?

5. Is there a manual? Is it easy to use? Cost?

6. Is there a tutorial? Is it easy to use? Cost?

7. Is there a quick reference guide? Is it easy to use? Cost?

8. Is there training? Is it at your site or vendor's site? Cost?

9. Is there software support? Cost?

10. Are there software upgrades available? Cost?

11. How many organizations currently use this software?

Here are steps to take when purchasing development software:

1. Review trade publications and request information on the eight to ten software packages that appeal to you the most.

2. Review literature, making comparison grids regarding cost, features, etc.

3. Talk with associates and friends who might know about development software. Ask them if you can have a demonstration of the software at their site, with their prime user.

4. Be wary of the person who promises to "build you a simple package and save you a lot of money."

5. Identify the top three packages you are interested in and set up demonstrations at your site. Include the executive director, director of development, office manager, information technology (IT) manager, and the person who will be the prime user. Be sure the person who knows everything about your development program in detail is part of the mix.

6. Know your equipment well enough to be aware of additional equipment you may require.

7. Ask a lot of questions during demonstrations.

8. Ask for references of people who use the package in your area and visit them. Ask a lot of questions.

9. Purchase a support package with upgrades.

10. Purchase off-site training. Make sure that your staff is well trained and knowledgeable about the software so it can be used to its maximum potential.

11. Stay on top of installation and ask questions throughout the process. If you have concerns, voice them immediately and get answers.

Know that no software package is perfect, and it takes time and energy to get your development office record-keeping system in place.

—*Karen Medicus*

Appendix D.8

Sample Direct-Mail Pieces

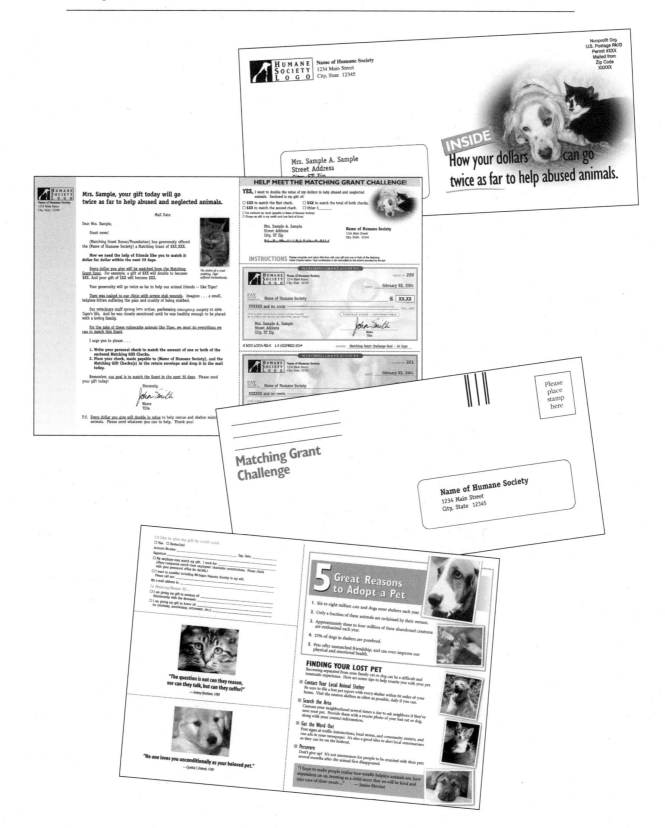

continued…

Help STOP Animal Cruelty

LOGO

"He who is cruel to animals becomes hard also in his dealings with men. We can judge the heart of a man by his treatment of animals." Immanuel Kant

Dear Ms. Sample,

Every year the Anywhere Humane Society takes in animals who need new homes. Lost, abandoned or abused, we provide the veterinary care, healthy meals and love these animals need. We have our hands full trying to care for them all -- our resources are stretched as it is.

That's why I've enclosed two reply slips and two reply envelopes. The first is for you to send a gift of $XX this month. Then I hope you will save the September reply slip and envelope and send another gift next month to help rescue and care for homeless and abused animals like Mandy.

A few days before we actually saw Mandy, we received a call from a concerned neighbor that there was a dog needing our help. She was concerned that the dog's owner had used inhumane methods to stop Mandy from barking.

It was a dreary day when we went to check on Mandy. From a distance, we could see that she was tied up outside with no food, water or shelter.

As we walked closer, Mandy looked at us with fear.

Our hearts sank when we got close enough to see that Mandy's mouth and nose were rubber-banded together so tightly that she could not bark. Sadly, Mandy's nose had been rubber-banded shut for so long that it was worn down to the skin. Mandy was also severely underweight.

Even though she was scared, Mandy seemed to understand that we were there to help.

We immediately removed Mandy and took her to the shelter for medical care, a good meal and a safe home.

(over, please)

Mandy stayed at the shelter for nearly two months during the time her owner was being prosecuted. The staff and volunteers watched Mandy come out of her shell in an environment full of love and care. We watched her grow to a healthier weight and were amazed at the love and personality she possessed, despite having been through so much trauma.

Mandy's story ends happily. Her owner was successfully prosecuted and Mandy was put up for adoption and placed in a new, loving home just two days later!

We know we can't help every single animal who needs us. But we will try. We open our doors to the animals who need temporary shelter and care while new, loving homes are found. We work to end the abuse and neglect that makes our shelter necessary.

But we can't do it without you. Every dollar you send helps us provide a second chance to more animals like Mandy. Please help us give them that chance.

Stories like this are what we are all about and why I hope you will support our efforts to "Stop Animal Cruelty."

Your generous gift will help us:

- Find new, loving homes for abandoned animals
- Provide veterinary care and medications for sick animals.
- Spay or neuter every dog and cat before it leaves our shelter.
- Work with police and prosecutors to ensure that those who commit the most serious animal abuse charges are prosecuted to the fullest extent of the law.

Please help us rescue animals from danger and indifference and give them the kind and loving treatment they deserve. Your gift will help us do all of this and more! Please think of Mandy and write the largest check you can.

Thank you!

n Smith
Executive Director

I've enclosed two reply forms and two envelopes -- one for August and one September. It would mean so much if you could use the August envelope for gift today, and then match that gift for September.

Non-Profit Org.
U.S. POSTAGE
PAID
PERMIT # xxx
Mailed From
Zip Code xxxxx

Help STOP Animal Cruelty

…before it's too late.

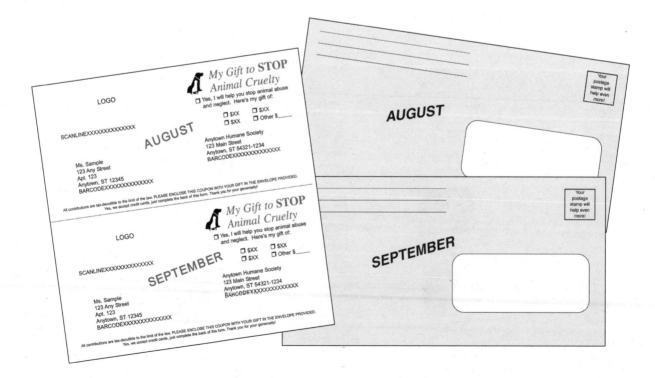

156

Fund-Raising for Animal Care Organizations

Name:
Gandalf

Age:
5 years

Before I came to the shelter I was living the rough life on the streets, terribly hungry and tormented by kids who would set my fur on fire. Good thing a nice lady intervened for me! Although she couldn't keep me herself she gave me some good food and then took me to the shelter where I had time to heal. Four months later I was adopted by a loving family with three very nice children and two friendly cats. I just love my new home, and hope that more lonely cats and dogs get a second chance like I did!

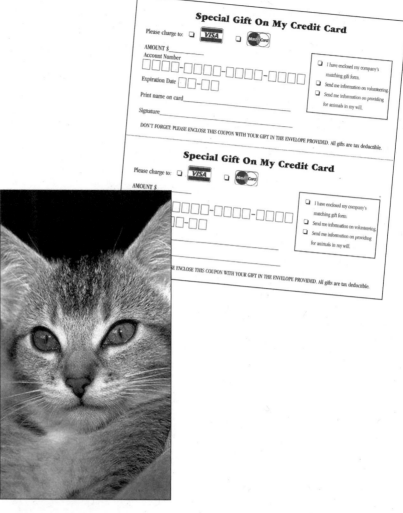

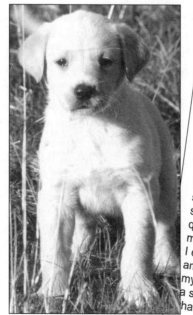

Name:
Atlas

Age:
4 months

I was surrendered with my mother by a backyard breeder who no longer thought we were convenient. Since the time I was born I had only negative contact with humans, and so was very scared when I first arrived at the shelter. My mother warmed up quickly to the staff but it is taking me a little longer to trust in them. I enjoy the snacks they give, but am still not sure if humans have my best interests in mind. I am in a special behavior program so that I can learn to trust, and be ready for adoption soon.

Appendix D.8 Sample Direct-Mail Pieces

Appendix D.9

Sample Special Events and Sample Budget

Sample Events

Dog Walk/Run

Dog walk/run events are popular special events for animal care organizations. After all, few other special events host the very creatures your organization was created to protect. With a dog walk/run event, the pledge is key to raising larger chunks of money. When no registration fee is required, participants "win" items only when they raise certain dollar amounts through pledges ("$50 in pledges gains you one T-shirt," for example). Even when participants pay a registration fee, they are still encouraged to collect pledges. Each method has advantages and disadvantages, so you need to decide which is best for your organization and target population.

House or Cocktail Party

Ask board members or other volunteers to host a gathering of their friends and colleagues at their home. They arrange for the meal (brunch, lunch, dinner, or appetizers) and ask each guest to make a small donation to your organization. During the event, your executive director, another staff person, or a board member talks about your organization's programs and relates success stories. The following day, send thank-you notes to all attendees. Be sure to add them to your mailing list to receive newsletters and direct-mail appeals (or, better yet, a personalized solicitation letter from the board member who invited them to their home.) Similar parties can be designed as cultivation events for major donors. Afterward, develop and implement a solicitation strategy for each attendee.

Silent or Live Auction

Soliciting, collecting, and organizing the items for an auction can be time-intensive. However, an auction done in conjunction with a dinner, cocktail party, or other special feature can add to the total raised. In a silent auction, bidders submit their bids on paper. Live auctions require a good auctioneer to get the bidding started and go as high as possible. Many agencies will combine a live auction of a few high-end items with a silent auction for the rest of the items.

One "item" you should never put up for bid is a live animal—not even a shelter animal available for adoption. If you want to include an adoption in your auction, stress that you are not auctioning off a specific animal but rather an opportunity to adopt (an adoption certificate, for example). Explain that this adoption will be of an animal that is appropriate for the winner and that you reserve the right to refuse an adoption that is not appropriate. Before including this type of auction item, carefully consider all the ethical and logistical issues. For example, what if the winner does not qualify? How will you compensate that person and soothe hurt feelings? How will you make the community understand the difference between auctioning an animal-adoption opportunity versus an actual animal adoption? Follow the lead of the Humane Society of Boulder Valley, whose written program and auctioneer clearly detailed such considerations at its "Puttin' on the Leash" event.

Baby Shower

(This is appropriate for those organizations with animal-fostering and adoption programs.) Designed to support a foster program, the event is best held during the summer when you have a lot of kittens and puppies. Set it up like a traditional baby shower: ask invited guests to bring gifts for the shelter babies: kitten and puppy food and/or formula, playpens, blankets, feeding bottles, heating pads, etc. In the invitation or at the event, ask guests to "sponsor" the babies (a single kitten for $50, a litter of puppies for $250, or whatever level works for your organization). At the event, you can engage attendees in games, lead a tour of the foster care area, give guests an opportunity to meet some fosterlings who are ready for adoption, and introduce some of your foster parent volunteers.

Benefit Dinner

These popular events come in many variations. A black-tie or awards event may be combined with a live or silent auction, a fashion show, a celebrity speech or performance, or musical entertainment. If your community already has a large number of benefit dinners, come up with some twist that will make yours stand out. Can you design one that allows people to bring their dogs? What about highlighting an animal art auction? These dinners (or brunches or lunches) typically offer ten-seat tables, each sold to corporate sponsors or major donors who invite friends to join them. You should offer several price levels, providing perks like ad space in the program and front-of-the-room seating for the higher-priced tables. In addition to selling tables, offer individual tickets. To meet fund-raising goals, it is important that your board members be willing to sell tables to their business colleagues and acquaintances.

Fashion Show

An animal care organization can hold a unique fashion show with both human and animal models. In most fashion shows, the clothing is lent by high-end stores. Consider asking a pet-supply store in an upscale shopping area to help with fashion accessories for your animal models—collars, leashes, jackets, beds for smaller pets—all simple items animals can model comfortably. Remember that yours is an animal care organization—that means no fur products!

No Ball/Non-event

The "no ball" or "non-event" is not really a special event—it is a creative direct-mail appeal. The thinking behind these "non-events" is that many people are happy to support your cause but are not particularly anxious to attend your event. For a non-event, you send invitations asking people to donate money for the privilege of not attending the nonexistent event. You can have some fun creating the "benefits" donors receive for the donation level they choose. For example, the $50 level may entitle the donor not to attend a "rubber chicken" dinner, and a $150 level may entitle the donor not to have to wear black tie. To cultivate major donors, consider holding a small reception for them at a private home or other exclusive location in conjunction with your non-event invitation mailing.

Art Show

Arrange for a group of local artists with animal-related art to do a benefit show from which a portion of the proceeds goes to your organization. The IRS does limit the deduction an artist can take for donated art to the cost of his supplies. So look into arranging the event so that your organization receives the portion that would normally go to the gallery or ask the artists to donate a percentage of anything sold.

Food-Wine-Beer Festival/Carnival/Street Fair

You have a lot of different options with street fair or festival special events. You can invite several area restaurants or breweries to participate or you can create a carnival event with some food vendors. To distinguish your event from others, look for a location where people can bring their pets. This type of event is designed to be a relatively high-volume, low-entry-fee event, so be sure that you can draw enough people to make the event profitable.

Calendar Contest

In calendar contests, people submit photos of their animals to compete for prominent placement in your organization's photo calendar. If you charge a fee for each entry submitted and guarantee placement in the calendar, the income will pay for the printing and production costs. (Most photos will end up in the photo collage pages, while the winning photos appear on "animal of the month" pages.) The entry fee may or may not include a free copy of the calendar. Calendars can be sold to raise additional revenue. If you have a good relationship (or can develop one) with a local sports team or other group of celebrities, consider producing a calendar featuring them with their pets. These types of calendars have been most successful when the sports team or other business sponsors the cost of the calendar and the proceeds from the sale benefit your organization.

Santa Photo

Offer people a chance to have their pets' picture taken with Santa. If your Pets-and-Santa photo event is held early enough (say in late October), participants can purchase sets of personalized photo holiday cards. You can sell different photo packages, such as photo only, photo holiday cards, and even photos on disk (if the photographer uses a digital camera).

Telethon

These live television events can be both labor-intensive and costly. To hold a telethon, you first need to find a local TV station willing to sell you the airtime for the event. Next you'll need to find a good producer to ensure the event's success. Sponsorships are solicited beforehand for different sets and segments of the show, and viewers are urged to call in with pledges during the show. Be sure to provide incentives for viewers to make their pledges on credit cards, which get you the money quickly and cut down on collection costs.

Raffle

People buy tickets for the chance to win prizes in a drawing. You can sell an unlimited number of tickets, usually at low cost and sometimes with a discount for multiple-ticket purchase (for example, $5 per ticket or six tickets for $25). Or you can sell a limited number of tickets at a high price, usually $100 or more. If you hold a raffle with a limited number of tickets, the prize needs to be something of great value, like a car or a vacation. Never offer an animal as a prize in your raffle, for the reasons mentioned earlier.

Flea Market/Garage Sale/Sale of Items

If your organization does not have a thrift store, consider holding a special event expressly to sell donated items. Such an event allows you to accept and sell donated items that you cannot use in your facility. The donations don't need to be animal-related.

Dog House/Cat Tree/Dog Bowl Art Auction

For this media-friendly event, you would invite well-known community members and celebrities to build a doghouse or cat tree or decorate a dog bowl, then sell these items at an auction. As an alternative, you can approach groups, such as homebuilders, to create the doghouses or cat trees.

Valentine's Day Event

Consider a Valentine's Day event inviting people to send in a photo and valentine for their pet. In exchange for an entry fee, the photo and valentine would be displayed for a week in your facility or at a local shopping center. An adoption event or other activity could kick off the display.

Spokesperson/Celebrity Contest

Invite people to enter their pet in a judged contest that selects a winner to serve as "spokes-animal" for your organization for a year. Charge a fee for each entry. Limiting entries to animals adopted from your organization would be a great opportunity to keep adopters involved.

Restaurant/Bar Benefit and "Dine Out for Dogs"

For this type of event, a local restaurant or bar hosts a benefit in which the evening's cover charges or a portion of the proceeds go to your organization. If the restaurant has an outdoor area where guests can sit with their dogs, you can promote the benefit as a "Dine Out with Your Pet" event. If you can get several restaurants to hold their benefit on the same evening, bill it as a "Dine Out for the Dogs" event.

Concert

Do you know a local band that supports your organization or an animal-loving musician scheduled to perform in your town? If so, see if you can schedule a benefit concert for your organization. Some concert promoters or professional athletic teams will offer discounted blocks of tickets that you can sell at the regular price and keep the difference for your organization.

Veggie Cook-off

In this event, cooks prepare a dish (vegetarian chili, spaghetti, soups, etc.) to be judged by the participants. Inviting local restaurant chefs can make this type of an event especially fun and competitive.

Singles Event with Dogs

Interested in drawing singles to a special event? Consider creating a special event just for them. If your organization is in an urban area with a substantial population of unattached people, invite them and their pets to a singles event such as a hike, walk, or party in a location that allows animals.

Awards Event

Awards events are often combined with benefit dinners. You can choose to recognize community members who contribute to animal welfare in your area, volunteers, staff, government officials, or businesspeople.

Reunion Event

Invite people who have adopted their pets from your organization to an event with the pets. You can target a special component of a walk or street fair to alumni.

Film Festival

Invite a local theater to hold a benefit screening of animal-related films for your organization.

Motorcycle Ride

Motorcycle groups frequently host rides that benefit nonprofit organizations. If you know people involved with one of these groups, see if they will host a ride benefiting your group. If you have a location that would make a good start, finish, or rest stop, use it as a way to get your message out to the riders and thank them for their support.

Rare "Dogs Allowed" Venue

Take a look at the contacts your organization has with people in the community and government. Can you get permission to "break the rules" for a one-time event with dogs in a "no dogs allowed" location—an especially nice park, the ballpark, an amusement park, a shopping center, or some other location? The opportunity to take your pets to a "no pets allowed" location can be a great draw for the event.

Barn Tour

Instead of house tours, offer barn tours.

Sample Budget

Possible Revenue Categories:

Sponsorships:
# of sponsors $ Level   Total $ Received

Ticket sales:
tickets sold $ Level   Total $ Received

Registration:
people registered $ Level   Total $ Received

Additional Pledges

Vendor Registration and Percentage of Sales

Program/Ad Booklet:
ads sold $ Level   Total $ Received

Additional Donations

Raffle or Auction Proceeds

Cash Bar

Possible Expenses:

Rental:
  Location
  Equipment
      (tables, chairs, canopies, plates, napkins, tablecloths,
      scaffolding, portatoilets, trash bins, etc.)

Audiovisual:
  Production
  Equipment rental

Printing:
  "Save the Date" cards
  Invitations
  Registration forms
  Posters
  Donor agreement forms
  Bid sheets
  Folders
  Programs
  Bib numbers
  Tickets
  Press packets

Postage and Mail house

T-shirts and Incentive Items

Entertainment Costs

Credit Card Fees

Advertising

Insurance

Licenses and Permits

Photography

Food and Supplies for Committee Meetings and Volunteer Training

Thank-you Gifts and Awards

Security

Miscellaneous

Complimentary Tickets

—Judy Calhoun

Appendix D.10

Sample Special Events Timeline

Sample Timeline
WALK/RUN EVENT—STAFF TIME LINE
Event scheduled for: Saturday, May 1, 2004

Task	Responsibility	Deadline
JULY/AUGUST 2003		
Conduct focus groups of past participants for input	Event Coordinator	August 31, 2003
Orientation for new committee members	All Staff	August 31, 2003
Subcommittee chairs in place	All Staff	August 31, 2003
Committee members in place	Event Coordinator	August 31, 2003
Budget in place	Event Coordinator	October 1, 2003
SEPTEMBER 2003		
Logo/artwork approved	All Staff	September 1, 2003
First committee meeting	Event Coordinator	September 1, 2003
Sponsor letter and video mailed to sponsors	Sponsorship Coordinator	September 30, 2003
Research and identify potential sponsors	All Staff	December 31, 2003
OCTOBER 2003		
Committee meeting	Event Coordinator	October 1, 2003
Review pledge levels and incentive gifts	Pledge Coordinator	October 31, 2003
Begin solicitation of new sponsors	Sponsorship Coordinator	December 31, 2003
Begin research of business for corporate teams	Corporate Team Coordinator	April 15, 2004
NOVEMBER 2003		
Committee meeting	All Staff	November 5, 2003
Review volunteer positions and job descriptions	Volunteer Coordinator and Key Staff	November 15, 2003
Obtain bids on pledge incentive gifts	Pledge Coordinator	November 30, 2003
Confirm parking facilities	Event Coordinator	November 30, 2003
Begin drafting brochure	Writer/Editor	December 1, 2003
Draft marketing plan	Marketing Coordinator	December 1, 2003
DECEMBER 2003		
Committee meeting	All Staff	December 3, 2003
Confirm registration sites	Registration Coordinator	December 15, 2003
Review brochure copy	Key Staff	December 15, 2003
Obtain bids on T-shirts	Pledge Coordinator	December 15, 2003

Fund-Raising for Animal Care Organizations

Task	Responsibility	Deadline
Order sponsor gifts	Sponsorship Coordinator	December 15, 2003
Develop equipment list	Event Coordinator	December 15, 2003
Order storage container	Event Coordinator	December 15, 2003
Finalize pledge incentive levels and gifts	Pledge Coordinator	December 30, 2003
Confirm major sponsors for brochure, poster, T-shirt	Sponsorship Coordinator	December 30, 2003

JANUARY 2004

Task	Responsibility	Deadline
Begin volunteer sign-ups	Volunteer Coordinator	January 1, 2004
Committee meeting	All Staff	January 7, 2004
Brochure design completed	Graphic Designer	January 10, 2004
Media release—save the date, corporate recruitment	Media Coordinator	January 15, 2004
Corporate team recruitment plan in place	Corporate Team Coordinator	January 15, 2004
Poster design completed	Graphic Designer	January 15, 2004
Pledge incentive items ordered	Pledge Coordinator	January 15, 2004
Develop plan for distribution of brochures and posters	Marketing Coordinator	January 15, 2004
T-shirts ordered	Event Coordinator	January 31, 2004
Order bib numbers	Event Coordinator	January 30, 2004

FEBRUARY 2004

Task	Responsibility	Deadline
Event schedule finalized	Event Coordinator	February 1, 2004
Park layout finalized	Event Coordinator	February 1, 2004
Final proof of brochure	All Staff	February 1, 2004
Committee meeting	All Staff	February 4, 2004
Web-site banner and registration information up loaded	Web Master	February 5, 2004
Brochure to printer	Graphic Designer	February 5, 2004
Poster to printer	Graphic Designer	February 10, 2004
Instructions and plan for registration data entry written	Registration Coordinator	February 15, 2004
Schedule volunteer orientation	Volunteer Coordinator	February 15, 2004
Event day equipment ordered (tables, chairs, canopies, scaffolding, portatoilets, trash containers, dumpsters, etc.)	Event Coordinator	February 15, 2004
Media release—web-site registration begins	Media Coordinator	February 15, 2004
Begin setting up appointments for corporate teams	Corporate Team Coordinator	February 15, 2004
Brochures mailed to past participants	Event Coordinator	February 28, 2004
Brochures and posters distributed throughout shelter	Event Coordinator	February 28, 2004
Begin distribution of posters and brochures	Marketing Coordinator	February 28, 2004

continued...

Task	Responsibility	Deadline
MARCH 2004		
Media release for April community calendars	Media Coordinator	March 1, 2004
Mail-in registration begins	Registration Coordinator	March 1, 2004
Storage container delivered	Event Coordinator	March 1, 2004
Committee meeting	All Staff	March 4, 2004
T-shirts delivered	Event Coordinator	March 5, 2004
Pledge incentive gifts delivered	Event Coordinator	March 5, 2004
Newsmagazine with brochure inserted mailed	Graphic Designer	March 10, 2004
Registration materials distributed to registration sites	Registration Coordinator	March 15, 2004
Meet with park staff to review plan	Event Coordinator	March 15, 2004
Newspaper and magazine ads designed	Graphic Designer	March 15, 2004
Arrange for security and police officers	Event Coordinator	March 31, 2004
Volunteer positions filled	Volunteer Coordinator	March 31, 2004
APRIL 2004		
Confirm schedule for volunteer orientation	Volunteer Coordinator	April 1, 2004
Volunteer confirmation letters sent	Volunteer Coordinator	April 1, 2004
Signage and banners ordered	Event Coordinator	April 1, 2004
TV/radio and newspaper PSAs run	Media Coordinator	April 1–April 30, 2004
Video/photo shot list developed	Media Coordinator	April 15, 2004
Sponsor thank-you letter drafted	Event Coordinator	April 15, 2004
Volunteer thank-you letter drafted	Volunteer Coordinator	April 15, 2004
Finalize event day plan and schedule	Event Coordinator	April 15, 2004
Mail-in registration ends	Registration Coordinator	April 20, 2004
Finalize equipment order	Event Coordinator	April 20, 2004
Volunteer orientation	Volunteer Coordinator	April 22, 2004
Pre-registration closes at 5 P.M.	Registration Coordinator	April 28, 2004
Web-site registration closes at 5 P.M.	Registration Coordinator	April 28, 2004
Load equipment	All Staff	April 29, 2004
Pre-registration data entry completed by noon	Registration Coordinator	April 30, 2004
All pre-registration reports completed by 5 P.M.	Registration Coordinator	April 30, 2004
Transport applicable equipment to park	All Staff	April 30, 2004
Set up external deliveries	Event Coordinator	April 30, 2004
Preliminary set up at park	All Staff	April 30, 2004

Task	Responsibility	Deadline
MAY 2004		
Event day	All Staff	May 1, 2004
Post-event web-page designed and posted	Graphic Designer	May 2, 2004
Sponsor thank-you note cards signed and sent	Event Coordinator	May 5, 2004
Event thank-you ad designed	Graphic Designer	May 5, 2004
Volunteer thank-you letters sent	Volunteer Coordinator	May 7, 2004
Sponsor photos ordered	Event Coordinator	May 7, 2004
All data entry completed	Registration Coordinator	May 15, 2004
JUNE 2004		
Event reports and demographics run	Registration Coordinator	June 1, 2004
Participant thank-you to printer	Event Coordinator	June 1, 2004
$250+ thank-yous in mail	Event Coordinator	June 1, 2004
Sponsor photos, gifts, etc., delivered	Sponsorship Coordinator	June 1, 2004
Follow-up committee meeting	All Staff	June 2, 2004
Video completed	Media Coordinator	June 15, 2004

Appendix D.11

Sample Special Events Volunteer Reminder Letter

Dear Canine Games Volunteer,

**Thank you for agreeing to volunteer to be a part of the 13th Annual Canine Games.
It is our biggest event of the year!** We again expect to host more than 600 dogs and thousands of people at this year's event. Please read the guidelines below and review the enclosed brochure so you are up to date on all of the details.

- **LOCATION:** The games are being held at Chinquapin Park, 3210 King Street in Alexandria (next to TC Williams High School).

- **PARKING:** Volunteers may park in_____parking lots.

PLEASE MARK THE FOLLOWING PRE-GAME DATES ON YOUR CALENDAR

SATURDAY,_____CAPTAINS/VOLUNTEERS MEETING [generally one week before the actual event, but may be earlier]. ALL captains and other volunteers, if possible, are asked to come to Chinquapin Park at_____a.m. for a meeting to see the layout of the field, learn where your event will be located, pick up instructions for your particular event, and receive general instructions on the Canine Games. The Special Events Committee will be available to answer any of your questions at this time.

THURSDAY,_____TRUCK LOADING [the Thursday immediately preceding the actual event]. We will be loading trucks at **6:00 p.m.** at the shelter, 4101 Eisenhower Avenue, with all of the equipment, props, fencing, and stakes required for each individual event, tents, coolers, cases of drinks, and other items to support the Canine Games. We need many strong backs to help with these heavy and/or bulky items.

FRIDAY,_____SET UP [the night before the actual event]. We would appreciate if you come to Chinquapin Park Friday evening at **6:30 p.m.** to assist with setup. We really need help staking and fencing each event as this saves us valuable time in the morning. We will have pizza and sodas for all, and we will give out Canine Games T-shirts at the end of setup.

GAME DAY CHECK-IN AT_____AM. We will be expecting you to be at Chinquapin Park at_____**a.m.** on Saturday,_____. **WHEN YOU ARRIVE AT THE PARK, YOU ABSOLUTELY MUST CHECK IN AT THE INFORMATION TENT BEFORE GOING TO YOUR ASSIGNED AREA!** Even if you are a veteran of the Games and know exactly what to do, you still **must** check in first and sign a liability waiver.

STAY UNTIL_____PM. We need you to stay until_____**p.m.** to assist with take-down and general cleanup. And if you really want to impress us, we could use help loading the truck at the park at the end of the Games and unloading the truck back at the shelter later that afternoon.

- **RAIN OR SHINE!** We have yet to cancel this event due to weather. Rain might actually be welcome if it continues to be this hot!

- **DRESS CODE/VOLUNTEER T-SHIRTS.** We have special Games T-shirts for our volunteers and ask that you wear them at the event. If you can come to the Friday night meeting, we will have T-shirts available then. You can also pick them up at the park the morning of the event. The dew will be heavy at that time of the morning and shoes tend to get very wet. Please dress accordingly. It is also recommended that you wear insect repellent and/or wear long pants to minimize mosquito bites.

- **ATTENTION!** We need your full attention. Please DO NOT bring your own pet to the Games, even if he/she was adopted from us. Also, DO NOT bring children to this event. **Volunteers are only accepted if they are age 16 or older.**

- **REFRESHMENTS.** Volunteers are welcome to check in at refreshments and grab a free soda and complimentary refreshments. We would like to be able feed all of our volunteers, but our pizza and pasta sales are some of the event's largest moneymakers. When pizza arrives, please give the public at least a half-hour to sell before asking for free pizza. Volunteers are NOT entitled to free pasta from Tempo Restaurant. At the end of the event, please help yourself to what is left over.

- **PLEASE BRING WATER.** We are again without a water buffalo this year. Please bring AT LEAST a one-gallon container of water with you on the day of the event. It is acceptable to bring tap water in a large, used container as this will be used for dog drinking water. We will have plenty of bottled water for humans.

- **RAFFLE TICKETS!** We have some fabulous prizes for our raffle drawing this year, including two tickets to a Washington Redskins game. We are asking all of our volunteers to try to sell at least ten raffle tickets, which you will find enclosed. The raffle tickets are $1 each. Please give the buyer one section of the ticket and send the other half back to us (before the Games), with the buyer's name, address, and phone number on it, with the appropriate amount of money. The winner will be selected at the Games; participants **do not** have to be present to win. Of course, if you are a really enthusiastic seller, we will be happy to send you more tickets to sell!

If you have any questions or concerns, please call_____.

Thank you so much for your support and enthusiasm!

Appendix D.12

Sample Special Events Plans

Distraction Dash

General Description:

This event will consist of two separate lanes, with a dog competing in each lane. Each dog's owner will be positioned at the finish line while volunteer handlers hold the dogs at the starting line. The dogs will be timed as they run to the finish line, encountering enticing distractions along the way.

Rules:

1. The dog must be on leash by the owner until the handler takes responsibility. At the time the owner unleashes the dog to walk to the finish line, the handler will leash the dog with a shelter leash until the event begins. When the timer yells, "ARE YOU READY?" handlers will remove leashes and hold the dog until the timer signals "GO."

NOTE: Knee cushions have been included for the handlers at the starting line. It is recommended, however, that you **TRY** to get the dog to sit at the starting line. This will minimize the amount of kneeling required, and because you are in a standing position, you will have greater control over the dog.

2. Dogs must remain in their own lanes.

3. Owners must be at finish lines to receive dogs. Owners may encourage their dogs in the race by calling and gesturing.

4. At the conclusion of the race, dogs must be put on leash immediately.

5. The recorders/timers will register the time and all pertinent information on the dog **AT THE CONCLUSION** of each race.

6. The judge/League has the final authority in determining the suitability of a dog to enter this competition. The judge/League has total discretion on this point, and the judge's/League's decision is final.

7. Dogs must remain in their own lanes. While it is preferable to have the lanes run simultaneously, if a situation presents itself, you may run a lane individually, i.e., a more aggressive dog who should not be side-by-side with a dog in the adjacent lane; a problem arising in one lane that holds up the start of the other lane; not enough contestants in line to fill both lanes; etc. Competing lanes add to the excitement of the event for all involved, but safety and keeping the lines moving also need to be considered. Use your best judgment.

8. Dogs may enter this competition twice but not in succession.

9. The three best times **for EACH of the two lanes** will be entered on the official Canine Games score sheets, resulting in a total of six best times.

10. The top three medal winners will be determined by the fastest times of those six best times.

Equipment:

NOTE: Remember how all equipment is packed/boxed and all fencing/stakes are bundled, so you can return them the same way after the event.

1. 275 feet of snow fencing
2. 38 stakes to hold snow fencing
3. sledgehammer
4. chalk liner
5. clippers
6. 150 plastic fasteners for fencing
7. name sign of the event

Split all remaining items between the two lanes.
8. 2 stopwatches
9. 2 clipboards, 4 pens
10. 2 sets of Official Canine Games score sheets
11. 4 leashes—2 at the starting line & 2 at finish line
12. 2 knee cushions for handlers at the starting line

(Items provided may vary slightly from the listing below.)
13. stuffed animals
14. old shoes
15. rubber toys
16. balls
17. 2 trash cans
18. milkbones

continued…

Pre-event preparation:

1. The event will measure 86 feet long by 20 feet wide (two racing lanes, each 10 feet wide), to include a Catch Area extending beyond the finish line. Using chalk liner, mark off entry line, starting line, and finish line. **NOTE: THE STARTING LINE IS INSIDE THE FENCED AREA, 6 FEET DOWN FROM THE ENTRY LINE.** In the event a dog tries to escape to reach its owner, the handler will have an enclosed area to capture the dog.

2. Put the stakes in the ground to delineate the perimeter of the event, the center line dividing the two racing lanes, and a "catch" area at the finish line. Attach snow fencing from post to post to separate the racing lanes, to form the perimeter, and to enclose the "catch" area. The "catch" fence is set up at the finish line, stretching approximately 10–15 feet beyond the end of the lanes. The stakes used for this area should be a minimum of 4 feet high to help contain the dogs. **Make a gate with the fencing and stakes for an exit for the owners and the dogs. There should be only ONE exit. THE CATCH AREA MUST BE TOTALLY ENCLOSED AND MUST ENCOMPASS BOTH LANES TO PREVENT LOOSE DOGS FROM ESCAPING.** One volunteer will man the gate to ensure that no dogs escape.

3. Using the chalk liner, mark off a line 15 feet from the event **STARTING LINE** to distance those waiting to compete so they do not affect the start of each race.

4. Scatter in each lane the stuffed animals, rubber toys, old shoes, balls, milkbones, turned-over trash cans, etc. (whatever is provided in your box). These may be in any order you choose.

5. Put the stake with the name sign for event into the ground.

6. Become familiar with operating the stopwatch.

7. Fill water bowls. Identify one person on the team to ensure that the water bowls are filled continuously.

NOTES:

1. The volunteers serving as the **timers/recorders should position themselves at the finish line.** The information pertinent to each contestant, such as the dog's number, name, etc., will be entered on the score sheet **AT THE END OF THE RACE**, along with the dog's time. This positioning saves the volunteer from having to run back and forth from the starting line to the finish line for each heat.

2. The timer/recorder will also act as a starter and signal, **"ARE YOU READY? GO!"** for each heat. AWLA leashes are provided for use in the catch area. Timers/recorders should be prepared to help catch loose dog in the event the owner is unable to leash his/her pet.

3. As the dog handler position can be demanding, the timers/recorders should rotate positions with the handlers throughout the competition.

4. Volunteer response permitting, a full-time assistant will be added, who will be shared among Distraction Dash and 2–3 other events. If you need a bathroom break, a break from your position, have equipment failure, etc., the assistant will be available to accommodate. He/she will make a continuous round between these events, which are close in proximity on the field. In addition, one field captain, who has been assigned to monitor your event and needs, will be making a continuous round throughout the competition.

Post event

1. Indicate the 1st-, 2nd-, and 3rd-place winners on the last page of the score sheets. **W R I T E   L E G I B L Y**.

2. Take the score sheets **IMMEDIATELY** to the **STAGE** and give them to one of the field captains.

3. Dismantle the event. **Repack all items, including the stakes, in the same packaging you received them.** Take all items to the Information Tent. Arrange the stakes and fencing in separate piles in one common area and put the event box(es) with the equipment all together in a separate common area AWAY FROM the stakes/fencing.

Personnel required:

1. Handlers—2 (one for each lane)

2. Timers/Recorders/Starters—2 (one person records and times each lane)

3. Shared Assistant—1

Total required: 4 Plus 1 Shared Assistant

Appendix D.13

Sample Pledge Form

Name _____

Home Address _____

City_____ State_____Zip_____

Home Phone _____ Work Phone _____

E-mail address _____

Employer_____

Employer Address _____

Employer City _____ State _____ Zip _____

To support the priorities of the Campaign, I (we) pledge the sum of $_____.

My (our) pledge will be payable in installments of $_____ over the next ____ years (we encourage pledges paid over 5 years), beginning _____, on the following schedule (check one):

   ❏ annually   ❏ semi-annually   ❏ quarterly   ❏ monthly

I (we) have enclosed a down payment of $ _____ (payment by check attached)

I would like to make a down payment via credit card:

   ❏ Visa   ❏ MasterCard   ❏ Discover   ❏ American Express

Account Number: _____ Expiration Date: _____

Name on the Card: _____

Would you like us to bill your credit card automatically on the schedule indicated above?

   ❏ Yes   ❏ No

Please list my (our) name(s) in all reports and on the Wall of Honor in the appropriate Giving Circle as:

_____

❏ I (We) wish to remain anonymous.

Signed: _____ Date: _____

Appendix D.14

Sample Confidential Donor Prospect Form

Name of referring party: _____

Address: _____

Home Phone: _____ Work Phone: _____

Prospective donor's name: _____

Address: _____

Phone: _____

Employer, if applicable: _____

Relationship to the referring party (if any):

    ❏ Relative

    ❏ Business associate

    ❏ Friend

    ❏ Contributor

    ❏ Other (please specify): _____

Why this individual might give to the campaign:

    ❏ Interested in the mission

    ❏ History of giving to similar institutions

    ❏ Previous contributions to the institution

    ❏ Other (please specify): _____

Most likely to make a five-year pledge of:

    ❏ $100,000 or more

    ❏ $50,000–$99,999

    ❏ $25,000–$49,999

    ❏ $10,000–$24,999

    ❏ $5,000–$9,999

    ❏ $1,000–$4,999

continued...

Can you get this individual to meet with you and another representative? ❒ Yes ❒ No

If not, how would you suggest making a contact with this individual? _____

_____

Other information known about this prospective donor that would be helpful, i.e., types
of charitable causes supported in the past, approximate net worth, special interests, desire
to be recognized for gifts, etc. _____

Date form completed: _____

Name of volunteer or staff member who solicited this prospect referral: _____

_____

Thank you!

Appendix D.15

Sample E-Newsletter

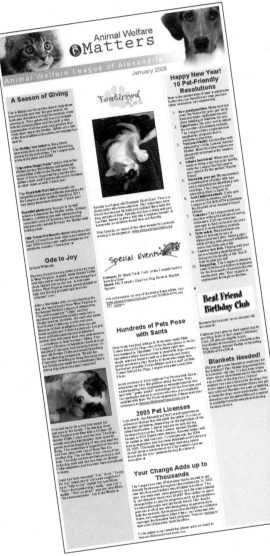

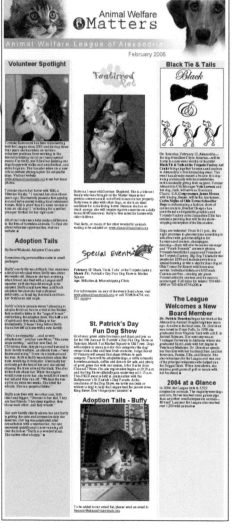

Resources

GENERAL FUND-RAISING INFORMATION

Organizations

American Humane Association
www.americanhumane.org
303-792-9900

American SPCA (ASPCA)
www.aspca.org
212-876-7700
www.imaginehumane.org
512-358-7005
(for fund-raising-specific inquiries)

**The Association of Fundraising
Professionals (AFP)**
www.afpnet.org
800-666-FUND

**The Humane Society
of the United States**
www.hsus.org
www.AnimalSheltering.org
202-452-1100

Humane Society University
www.humanesocietyu.org
www.hsuonline.org
301-548-7731

Nonprofit Risk Management Center
www.nonprofitrisk.com
202-785-3891

Books

Flanagan, J. 1999. *Successful fundraising: A complete
handbook for volunteers and professionals.* New York:
McGraw-Hill.

Herman, M., and D. Kirschbaum. 1999. *No strings
attached: Untangling the risks of fundraising and
collaboration.* Washington, D.C.: Nonprofit
Risk Management Center.

Keegan, P. 1990. *Fundraising for nonprofits: How
to build a community partnership.* New York:
HarperCollins Publishers, Inc.

Klein, K. 2001. *Fundraising for social change.*
San Francisco: Jossey-Bass.

Mutz, J., and K. Murray. 2000. *Fundraising for
dummies.* New York: Wiley Publishing, Inc.

Rosso, H., and Associates. 1991. *Achieving excellence
in fund raising.* San Francisco: Jossey-Bass.

Articles

Brown, B. 1999 (rev. 2003). *Getting your paws
on more money: Overcoming fundraising phobia.*
Best Friends Animal Sanctuary.

Lawson, N. Fundraising in the face
of uncertainty and loss. *Animal
Sheltering,* January–February 2002.
www.AnimalSheltering.org.

Web Sites

www.afpnet.org

www.allianceonline.org

www.boardsource.org

www.charitychannel.org

www.guidestar.org

www.independentsector.org

www.irs.gov

www.mapnp.nonprofitoffice.com

www.nonprofitnews.org

www.raise-funds.com

TOPIC-SPECIFIC RESOURCES

Market Research and Niche Development

Books

Andreasen, A. 2002. *Marketing research that won't break the bank.* San Francisco: Jossey-Bass.

Troughton, B., and C. Ginsberg. 2003. *Making plans to make a difference: Business planning for shelters to inspire, mobilize, and sustain change.* New York: American SPCA.

Articles

Savesky, K. 1999. Selling your organization's messages. *Animal Sheltering,* January–February. *www.AnimalSheltering.org.*

Web Sites

http://www.allianceonline.org/FAQ/strategic_ planning/how_can_we_do_competitive.faq (The MacMillan Matrix)

www.cbsm.com (community-based social marketing)

www.mapnp.org/library/research/research.htm (basic business research methods, management assistance program for nonprofits)

www.marketingprofs.com/tutorials/kanzler1.asp (positioning statement tutorial)

www.nichecraft.com ("Finding your niche," Lynda Falkenstein)

Ethical and Legal Resources

Giving USA Update

Annual survey of state laws regarding charitable solicitations. AAFRC Trust for Philanthropy. Available for purchase online at *www.aafrc.org.*

State Registration and Forms

www.multistatefiling.org

IRS Regulations

(IRS publications, available online at *www.irs.gov*):

Publication 526, *Charitable Contributions*

Publication 557, *Tax-Exempt Status for Your Organization*

Publication 561, *Determining the Value of Donated Property*

Publication 1771, *Charitable Contributions— Substantiation and Disclosure Requirements*

Publication 4221, *Compliance Guide for 501(c)(3) Tax-Exempt Organizations*

Maryland Nonprofits Standards for Excellence Program

www.standardsforexcellence.org

Ethics Tests

www.ephilanthropy.org
www.ethics.org
www.ftc.gov/charityfraud

Operation Phoney Philanthropy

www.ftc.gov/charityfraud

Prospect Research

Internet Tools

Biographical Information -Locating Prospects

www.555-1212.com
www.anywho.com
www.infospace.com
www.rootsweb.com
www.switchboard.com

Executive

www.ceoexpress.com
www.hoovers.com
www.tenkwizard.com

Lawyers

www.findlaw.com
www.martindale.com

News Sites

www.bizjournals.com
www.newslink.org
www.northernlight.com
www.prnewswire.com

Hard Assets—Real Estate

http://indorgs.virginia.edu/portico/assessors.html
http://realestate.yahoo.com/re/homevalues

Hard Assets—Insiders

www2.marketwatch.com/tools/quotes/insiders.asp
www.tenkwizard.com

Hard-Asset Sites—Salary Guides

www.jobsmart.org
www.salary.com

Hard-Asset Sites—Rich Lists

www.forbes.com/richlist
www.pathfinder.com/fortune

Hard Assets—Business Public Company

www.hoovers.com
www.sec.gov

Private Company

www.business.com
www.dnb.com
www.sos.state.tx.us/corp/sosda/index.shtml

Soft Assets— Foundation Affiliations

www.fdncenter.org
www.guidestar.com

Political Affiliations

www.tray.com/fecinfo

Other Web Resources

www.afpnet.org
www.aprahome.org
www.boardsource.org
www.idealist.org
www.indorgs.virginia.edu/portico
www.prospectinfo.com

Books

Marquis *Who's who: Who's who in America.* (Updated annually.) New Providence, N.J.: Marquis Who's Who.

Online Search Assistance

www.dowjones.com (major financial resources such as the *Wall Street Journal*, the *New York Times*, and *Barron's*)

www.knightridder.com (a collection of databases with a searchable index)

www.KnowX.com (business information reports on private companies)

www.lexisnexis.com (property holdings and Secretary of State records throughout the United States)

Direct Mail

Organizations

The Direct Marketing Association (DMA)
www.the-dma.org
212-768-7277

Grizzard
http://nonprofit.grizzard.com
800-241-9351

Mal Warwick & Associates
www.malwarwick.com
510-843-8888

The U.S. Post Office
www.usps.com/directmail

National Association of Attorneys General
www.naag.org

Foundations and Grant Proposals

Books

Barber, D. 1994. *Finding funding: The comprehensive guide to grant writing.* Long Beach, Calif.: Bond Street Publishers.

Collins, S. 2003. *The Foundation Center's guide to winning proposals.* New York: Foundation Center.

Golden, S. 1997. *Successful grantsmanship: A guerilla guide to raising money.* San Francisco: Jossey-Bass.

Hall, M. 2003. *Getting funded: A complete guide to proposal writing.* Portland, Ore.: Portland State University Continuing Education Publications.

Web Sites

www.cof.org
www.fdncenter.org
www.guidestar.org

Planned Giving

Organizations and Companies

National Committee on Planned Giving
www.ncpg.org
317-269-6274

R & R Newkirk
www.rrnewkirk.com
800-342-2375

Robert F. Sharpe & Co.
(The Sharpe Group)
www.sharpenet.com
800-238-3253

Stelter Company
www.stelter.com
800-331-6881

Books

Ashton, D. 2004. *The complete guide to planned giving.* Quincy, Mass.: Ashton Associates.

Maple, S. 2002. *The complete idiot's guide to wills and estates.* New York: Alpha Books.

Seltzer, M. 2001. *Securing your organization's future.* New York: The Foundation Center.

Sharpe, R. 1999. *Planned giving simplified: The gift, the giver, the gift planner.* New York: John Wiley and Sons, Inc.

Articles

Derek, D. 2001. The future of planned giving: Seniors and the online revolution. *Fundraising Management*: 32 (April).

Johnson, B. 2002. Let's talk about planned giving. *Grassroots Fundraising Journal* 21: 2.

Schackmann, R. Is your nonprofit walking away from money? *http://nonprofit.grizzard.com/articles.cfm*.

Schmeling, D. 1998. The "why" of planned giving. *Grassroots Fundraising Journal* 17: 6.

———. 1999. Marketing planned giving. *Grassroots Fundraising Journal* 18: 1.

———. 1999. Budgeting for planned giving. *Grassroots Fundraising Journal* 18: 3.

Zachar, H. The seven keys to success in planned giving. *http://nonprofit.grizzard.com/articles.cfm*.

Web Sites

www.charitychannel.com
(model gift policy manual)
www.hsus.org/pets/pet_care/providing_for_your_pets_future_without_you
www.pgdc.com/usa
www.pgtoday.com
www.plannedgivingpulse.com

Special Events

Books

Freedman, H., and K. Feldman. 1998. *The business of special events: Fundraising strategies for changing times.* Sarasota, Fla.: Pineapple Press, Inc.

Klein, K. 2001. *Fundraising for social change.* San Francisco: Jossey-Bass.

Stallings, B., and D. McMillan. 1999. *How to produce fabulous fundraising events.* Pleasanton, Calif.: Building Better Skills.

Wendroff, A. 1999. *Special events: Proven strategies for nonprofit fund raising.* New York: John Wiley and Sons, Inc.

Articles

Albrecht, K. and C. Carman. 2003. The evolution of a special event. *Grassroots Fundraising Journal* 22: 6.

Association of Fundraising Professionals. 2001. What's up with special events. *Advancing Philanthropy*, July/August.

Harrison, B. 1997. Charitable organizations' special events. *Fund Raising Management*, July.

Metzger, G. 2003. After the lights go out. *Grassroots Fundraising Journal* 22: 4.

Wong, R. 2002. Special events issue. *Grassroots Fundraising Journal* 21: 6.

———. 2003. Tips on working with special events consultants. *Grassroots Fundraising Journal* 22: 4.

Online Fund-Raising

Books

Hecht, B., and R. Ramsey. 2002. *ManagingNonprofits.org: Dynamic management for the digital age.* New York: John Wiley and Sons, Inc.

Warwick, M., T. Hart, and N. Allen. 2002. *Fundraising on the Internet: The ePhilanthropyFoundation.org's guide to success online.* San Francisco: Jossey-Bass.

Articles

Derrico, K., and C. Allen. 2001. Clicking for dollars. *Animal Sheltering*, September–October. *www.AnimalSheltering.org.*

Web Sites

www.bcentral.com
www.cmarket.com
www.ephilanthropy.org
www.networkforgood.org
www.nonprofitnews.org
www.selfpromotion.com
www.techsoup.org
www.trafficmagnet.net
www.volunteermatch.org